Women, AIDS, and Activism

Women, AIDS, and Activism

by
The ACT UP/New York
Women and AIDS Book Group

Marion Banzhaf, Cynthia Chris (coeditor), Kim Christensen,
Alexis Danzig, Risa Denenberg, Zoe Leonard,
Deb Levine, Rachel Lurie, Monica Pearl (coeditor),
Catherine Saalfield, Polly Thistlethwaite,
Judith Walker, and Brigitte Weil

SOUTH END PRESS   BOSTON, MA

Acknowledgments

We thank Loie Hayes and South End Press for their commitment and assitance. We also thank ACT UP/New York for its support and financial help. Additionally, we thank the several women who made donations to this project from the settlement of a lawsuit prompted by the illegal strip-search of 29 ACT UP women after our demonstration at City Hall in March 1989.

The original Women and AIDS Handbook Group was Marion Banzhaf, Amy Bauer, Kim Christensen, Alexis Danzig, Risa Denenberg, Heidi Dorow, Zoe Leonard, Deb Levine, Maria Maggenti (editor), Ellen Neipris, Ann Northrop, Sydney Pokorney, Karen Ramspacher, Polly Thistlethwaite, Maxine Wolfe, and Brian Zabcik.

Cover and text design by Torry Colichio
Text production by Sheila Walsh and the South End Press collective
Printed in the U.S.A. on acid-free paper

Cover photo by Susie Silbar: An April 1990 Chicago demonstration resulting in the admission of women to the AIDS Unit of Cook County Hospital

Library of Congress Cataloguing-in-Publication Data
Women, AIDS, and Activism / by the ACT UP/NY Women
and AIDS Book Group : Marion Banzhaf ... [et al.].
    p.   cm.
Includes bibliographical references and index.
ISBN 0-89608-394-2 : $25.00 -- ISBN 0-89608-393-4 (pbk) : $7.00
1. AIDS (Disease) -- Social aspects. 2. AIDS (Disease) -- Political aspects. 3. Women -- Diseases. I. Banzhaf, Marion. II ACT UP (Organization) / NY Women and AIDS Handbook Group.
RC607.A26W65   1990
362.1'9697'92 -- do20

98 97 96 95 94 93 92 91 90   1 2 3 4 5 6 7 8 9
South End Press, 116 Saint Botolph Street, Boston, MA 02115

TABLE OF CONTENTS

Preface

This book was originally produced by members of the Women's Caucus of the AIDS Coalition to Unleash Power (ACT UP) in conjunction with a teach-in about women and AIDS at the Lesbian and Gay Community Services Center in New York City in March 1989. Our primary objectives in revising the text for publication were to advance research by and about women in the AIDS crisis, provide information about women's particular needs, analyze the impact of AIDS on women's lives from a feminist perspective, and promote grassroots activism.

Producing this book has revealed how little is known about women and HIV infection, and how scattered the information is. The book reflects eight months of exhaustive research on existing studies and their failures to consider all the issues in women's lives, and to connect women with existing resources for people with AIDS. We realized that different questions needed to be asked. in order to establish future research priorities, to identify women's treatment issues, to make demands for change in the health care system, and to overcome the barriers to fighting HIV infection. We challenge assumptions about how women are affected by HIV infection and fight the invisibility of women in the AIDS crisis.

This book is the result of a true collective process. Many women contributed their time and energy. Many women from outside the ACT UP/NY Women and AIDS Book Group contributed essays. We sought a number of these contributions because the group, as white women and Jewish women, could not represent all women. This book would not be complete without the perspectives of HIV-positive women, women with AIDS, and women of color involved in fighting the AIDS crisis. Several women contributed accounts of their experiences fighting the many oppressions that interconnect in the AIDS crisis. We provide the following information and analyses in the hope that it will spark others to begin organizing and taking action around issues concerning women and AIDS.

ACT UP! FIGHT BACK! FIGHT AIDS!

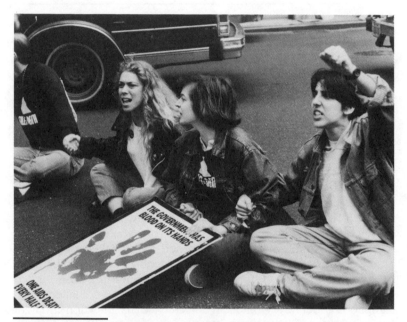

ACT UP demonstration "Wall Street II" in March 1988 marking ACT UP's second birthday and protesting the lack of money spent on AIDS.

Photo by Miriam Lefkowitz

What the Numbers Mean

RISA DENENBERG

Why do women die from AIDS so much faster than do men? Why are so many women with HIV illness of African descent or Latina? Why is the research on women with HIV disease so limited? How can we understand what all the statistics mean?

Numbers can be alarming but also revealing. In order to get answers, we need to ask the right questions and take a hard look at the available data. The growing number of women with HIV disease parallels a rise in cancer, drug use, homelessness, incarceration, and poverty among women.

Epidemiology is the science that studies epidemics and describes the occurrence and distribution of disease in a given location or population. Its goals include explaining how a particular disease is affecting people, how it is transmitted (passes from person to person), and how it can be prevented or controlled.

In the United States it is estimated that health care workers report 80 to 90 percent of all AIDS cases to local health departments, who then report them to the Centers for Disease Control (CDC). The CDC places each case in a category of exposure (the way the person is presumed to have gotten the virus) and generates statistics and predictions based on these data. In August 1989, the number of AIDS cases reported to the CDC reached 100,000.

While the number of AIDS cases is monitored, the number of people who are HIV positive is only estimated. The U.S. Public Health Service estimates that 1 to 1.5 million people are HIV positive at present. An international estimate from data collected by the World Health Organization suggests that 5 to 10 million people worldwide have been exposed to HIV. Many people who are HIV positive are well and may never get AIDS.

With a world view, epidemiologists have suggested that there are three distinct patterns of HIV transmission geographically. In pattern type I (which includes the United States, some western European countries, some Central American countries, Canada, New Zealand, and some countries in southern Africa) cases are disproportionately male (10 to 15 male cases for each female case), and perinatal transmissions (from woman to fetus during pregnancy and delivery) are low. In pattern II (including many central, eastern, and some southern African countries, and most of the Caribbean) the ratio of male to female cases is approximately equal, as are transmission rates from male to female and female to male. Perinatal transmission is high. Pattern III includes countries where there have been relatively few AIDS cases to date (including eastern Europe, northern Africa, much of Asia, and the Middle East).

The interval between diagnosis of AIDS and death from AIDS varies in different populations and may have to do directly with access to health care services. Survival times are shorter in African and Caribbean countries than they are in the United States. The little data we do have show clearly that in the United States survival times for women are shorter than those for men. Worldwide this means that people of color, poor people, and especially poor women of color are dying faster.

The number of AIDS cases in U.S. women reported to the CDC was 10,611 as of December 1989, representing 9 percent of the 117,781 cases. This represents a steady increase in the percentage of women diagnosed over the years of data collection (3 percent in 1981, 6.8 percent in 1983, and 9 percent in 1989). The geographic distribution is similar to that for men—New York, California, Florida, and New Jersey being the states with the greatest numbers of both men and women diagnosed with HIV.

The CDC has constructed a hierarchy of exposure categories. For example, a gay man who has had a blood transfusion would be recorded as exposed by homosexual/bisexual contact because it is listed first in the hierarchy. A bisexual woman who has sex with a gay man would be listed as exposed by heterosexual contact. And a lesbian intravenous drug user would be categorized as exposed by her IV drug use. This system assumes likelihood of transmission based on a U.S. model where AIDS was seen first in gay men. It does not list woman-to-woman contact as an exposure category and is probably inadequate to explain all the modes by which women get HIV. In the period from January 1989 to December 1989, the CDC listed women as having been exposed to HIV by intravenous (IV) drug use (52 percent), heterosexual contact (31 percent), receipt of blood transfusion (10 percent), and unknown (7 percent). The category of homosexual/bisexual contact, which accounts for 67 percent of men listed, excludes women. The next most numerous categories in men are intravenous drug use (18 percent), combined risk of IV drug use and homosexual/bisexual contact (8 percent—another category that applies only to men), heterosexual contact (3 percent), receipt of blood transfusion (2 percent), and unknown (3 percent). The most significant difference in the statistics for women is that the rate of unknown causes is more than double for women what it is for men. This highlights the concern that transmission of HIV in U.S. women is not fully understood.

A significant trend is the rapidly increasing rates of heterosexual transmission in women (any contact with a man is considered heterosexual, regardless of the man's sexual identity). These rates increased from 14 percent in 1982 to 17 percent in 1984, to 26 percent in 1986, and to 31 percent in 1989.

Ethnicity statistics for women, as of December 1989, break down as follows: Black (52 percent), white (27 percent), Latina (20 percent), Asian (0.6 percent), and Native American (0.24 percent). Seventy-three percent of women with AIDS are women of color, while 40 percent of men with AIDS are men of color (the U.S. population is approximately 25 percent people of color).

Epidemiological statistics do not account for all AIDS cases. An AIDS diagnosis is made after meeting the CDC's definition of AIDS, which was developed from the infections first observed in gay men in the United States in 1981. It was revised in 1985 and 1987, but is still based on the infections that gay men get. In brief, AIDS is diganosed in an HIV-positive individual when a predetermined set of unusual (opportunistic) infections or cancers are discovered and can be medically documented or when either a wasting syndrome (large weight loss) or HIV dementia (change in mental alertness) are identified. Rarely, an AIDS diagnosis will be conferred on an individual who is not HIV positive if one of the opportunistic infections or cancers associated with a compromised immune system is diagnosed definitively. HIV-positive people may be quite ill for months or years before meeting the definition of AIDS.

Since the CDC definition for AIDS was developed from observations of men, women often die of an opportunistic infection before they are even considered eligible for an actual AIDS diagnosis. Women are thus excluded from the total statistical picture. They not only won't get counted, they also won't get treated; they won't qualify for health benefits, child care, rent subsidies, or other support services

PWAs (People with AIDS) and AIDS activists have pressured the government to provide, and they won't be provided with information on how to take care of themselves and how to protect the people with whom they are having sex or sharing needles. Statistics, in other words, only count women who already fit into the CDC's narrow definition for AIDS; all the other women just remain invisible. Many women (and of course there are no statistics for this) are diagnosed with HIV infection only after they have died.

There are many questions that could be answered by epidemiologists that would promote a better understanding of women and AIDS. Woman-to-woman transmission must be studied, and homosexual/bisexual exposure categories must include women (of all sexual identities) who have been exposed to HIV through contact with gay and bisexual men. For men as well as for women, unknown exposure categories must be investigated, and a better understanding of the risks associated with specific sexual acts must be reached. The information currently available certainly suggests that more women are at risk in the United States than has been previously projected. The rising number of women with AIDS is alarming and must be heeded by activists, researchers, and public policymakers. The lives of women who are already ill and those who may be at risk depend on a greater understanding and a more effective response to women's experience of AIDS.

How Do Women Live?

KIM CHRISTENSEN

The impact of the AIDS crisis differs dramatically in various communities. Differing access to medical information, early interventions, and treatment, and differing abilities to take time off to take care of oneself, combine to make HIV infection a radically different experience for a wealthy, white, childless man than for a low-income Latina mother. HIV infection tends to worsen already existing forms of inequality and oppression based on gender, race and ethnicity, class, sexual orientation, and ability/disability level.

In order to understand the impact of the AIDS crisis on women, we need a realistic picture of where women are economically, politically, and medically in the United States today. Any group's access to resources, public attention, and power is critical in determining how well they fare in the AIDS epidemic.

Compared with men, women enter the AIDS crisis with fewer resources and support systems, and yet are responsible for more people. Our greater vulnerability to rape, battering, and other forms of sexual violence not only directly increases our chances of contracting HIV, but also places women in an inferior "bargaining position" when negotiating for safer sex.

The medical establishment's view of men as "the norm" further complicates HIV prevention, detection, and treatment for women. On the one hand, women are often invisible to medical researchers, and the AIDS research establishment is no exception. For example, many experimental AIDS drug trials completely exclude women. On the other hand, women are often treated as potential "fetus incubators" whose reproductive capacities are valued more than our lives, or as guinea pigs for the latest hormonal or surgical intervention. The traditional invisibility and powerlessness of women vis-à-vis the medical establishment mean that thousands of women are dying of

AIDS before a doctor even recognizes that our symptoms are related to HIV infection. Our inferior social status also makes it unlikely that treatments will be developed with our needs in mind.

Heterosexism, racism, and sexism are perhaps the three main forces that have fostered government inaction and allowed AIDS to reach pandemic proportions in the United States today. This chapter paints a statistical picture of U.S. women's current economic, political, and medical position. We need this foundation if we are to plan and organize actions that successfully address women's specific needs in the AIDS crisis.

Sexism and Women's Position in the AIDS Crisis

Sexist attitudes have had an enormous impact on the treatment of women in the AIDS crisis by the medical profession, public policy officials, and even some AIDS activists. Even more important than sexism—a set of bigoted attitudes about gender—has been the institution of patriarchy, which perpetuates male control over women's labor time, sexuality, and reproductive capacities. This male control may be exercised by an individual man, as in the case of a battering husband, or by male-dominated institutions, such as the Supreme Court, Congress, the New York Stock Exchange, the governing bodies of any of the major religions, or the medical profession.

Violence against women, including legal/societal toleration of this violence, is one of the most blatant aspects of patriarchal oppression. One out of three women in the United States will be raped during her lifetime.[1] The figures are even higher for African-American and Latina women.[2] Yet, because of the horrendous treatment raped women receive from police and medical authorities, less than ten percent of women who are raped report the crime.[3] Forty percent of all American wives are battered at some time in the course of their marriages.[4] The vast majority of women working outside of the home report being sexually harassed at least once on the job.[5] Reliable estimates of sexual abuse range from one-tenth to one quarter of all female children.[6]

Women learn very early that violence can be the price for "stepping out of line," for insisting on our opinions, our right to unrestricted mobility, our choice of dress or profession. This violence (and the constant *threat* of such violence) constricts our actions, reduces our aspirations, and distorts our self-images. A woman's exposure to HIV, and her ability to take care of herself if she becomes ill, may be largely determined by her exposure to male violence and the social supports she can use to defend herself.

Women's inferior economic status is another fundamental aspect of patriarchy. While women's participation in the paid labor force has increased by over 20 percent in the past three decades,[7] women's wages have not risen comparably. For example, white women who worked full time in 1988 earned about 65 percent of what white male full-time workers did.[8] Black and Latina women's incomes are even lower than those of white women, averaging 59 percent of what white men make.[9]

While women's earnings are generally two-thirds of men's, women are often responsible for more dependents. More than half of all marriages with children now end in divorce;[10] women get child custody in the vast majority of the cases;[11] only 23 percent of divorced mothers receive any child support payments at all;[12] and for those lucky enough to receive child support, the average amount is only $1,200 per year.[13] Many women, especially women with children, have to be financially dependent on men—either an individual man (father, husband, ex-husband, etc.) or the male-dominated state. The alternative, for many women and their children, is grinding poverty.

In the context of the AIDS crisis, women's inferior economic status means that we are less likely than men to have health insurance, less likely to be able to afford the consistent and high-quality medical attention necessary for early detection of HIV infection and opportunistic infections, and less likely to be able to afford quality treatment for ourselves and our children. For example, AZT, the only antiviral drug currently approved by the Food and Drug Administration for HIV infection, can cost up to $8,000 per year.[14] Since this is almost half of the average U.S. woman's annual earnings, it is unlikely that the many women without health insurance can afford it.

Since we live in a patriarchal society, women bear disproportionate responsibility for household labor and child care. A full-time working woman performs an average of 35 hours of physical housework labor per week, in addition to her 40-hour paid job.[15] The average woman who does not work outside the home performs 55 hours of such labor per week, more if she has more than two children.[16] The average husband and father performs less than a third of that labor time, which does not increase when his wife gets a paid job.[17]

This labor, although vital to the continued smooth functioning of the economy and the society, is not calculated as "work," nor does it count as part of the GNP. It does not provide the woman with health insurance, Social Security, or any independent income. Shouldering the burdens of the "double day" significantly reduces women's time for (among other things) basic self-care activities such as exercise and rest.[18] For an HIV-positive woman with children, this lack of self-care time can significantly reduce life expectancy.

Patriarchy also ensures women's lack of control over our sexuality and our reproductive capacities. In 1990, there is still no 100 percent effective and safe method of birth control. The tiny percentage of medical research devoted to this project speaks volumes about this society's lack of respect for women's health and autonomy, not to mention sexual pleasure. The medical establishment abhors the idea of experimenting on the male reproductive system, despite its being physically less complex and more accessible. It displays no such aversion to hormonal and other experimentation on women, particularly women of color in the United States, and women in the Third World.[19]

Increasing state control over abortion in the wake of the Supreme Court's 1989 *Webster* decision, combined with increasing forced abortion and sterilization of HIV-positive women (overwhelmingly women of color), threatens to steal away the fragile gains in control over reproduction for which women fought so hard in the 1960s and 1970s. In addition, lesbians encounter enormous obstacles in obtaining alternative insemination, in adopting or providing foster care for children, and in retaining custody of their biological children in cases of contested custody.

Reproductive freedom must mean real freedom of choice for lesbians, poor women, HIV-positive women, and women of color to avoid or terminate unwanted pregnancies, as well as to have or adopt children, to retain custody, and to raise them in safe and economically viable environments.

Control over sexuality and sexual choices is impossible without accurate information. Unfortunately, the majority of U.S. youth still do not receive sex education that is nonjudgmental regarding sexual choices and that deals with AIDS in a medically accurate way. Heated controversies have taken place in numerous school districts over informing students about condom use or distributing condoms, despite the fact that 70 percent of high school students are sexually active.[20]

In addition, the "double standard" for male and female sexuality is unfortunately still alive and well, with young women being held responsible for "controlling" and "harnessing" male sexuality, and for both birth control and safer sex negotiations. Yet all of the inequalities cited above (the threat of violence, economic dependence, etc.) often make negotiating sex, including safer sex, problematic for young women in heterosexual relationships.

The institutional supports for heterosexuality, and the threat of discrimination and violence against women who choose to express their lesbian sexuality, make "compulsory" heterosexuality the norm in the United States today. No woman can have sexual autonomy until she has the option of freely, and without fear, choosing to be sexual with another woman.

The dominant media bring patriarchal ideas and imagery into every U.S. household: from the virtual invisibility of lesbianism, to the romanticized sexual violence in scores of major films, to the absence of discussion of most of the major issues affecting women's lives.

Heterosexism is often used (in the media and by individual men) to reinforce sexism, and to scare heterosexual women into traditional sex roles. (For example, women in nontraditional occupations, or women who aggressively pursue our rights, are often called "dykes," regardless of their actual sexual orientations.) Sexist and heterosexist ideas and imagery serve to rationalize, perpetuate, and render invisible the physical, economic, sexual, and political oppression of women. They also make women, especially lesbians, almost totally invisible in the AIDS crisis.

Oppressed not just by patriarchy and sexism, most HIV-positive women are also subjected to racism, class oppression, heterosexism, and ableism. To draw an accurate picture of women's status, we need to examine briefly these forms of oppression.

Racism and AIDS

White supremacy is a set of institutions (supported by a set of racist ideas) that ensures that white people continue to have access to the labor and other resources of the various communities of color. Political, economic, and cultural control of these communities is often necessary for this to occur. Violence against people of color and official tolerance of and/or initiation of such violence remain institutionalized practices that perpetuate racism. Violence against people of color is not only perpetrated by young white men on the street, it also reaches into the highest levels of our government. For example, despite undisputed statistical evidence that a Black person is four times as likely to receive the death penalty as a white person convicted of a similar crime, the U.S. Supreme Court found that the death penalty is "not inherently racist" and does not violate the equal protection provisions of the Fourteenth Amendment.[21]

The U.S. government's drug policy is yet another example of institutional racism. Despite the "just say no" rhetoric, the government has tolerated and often actively participated in the flooding of communities of color with addictive drugs. This strategy was widely employed in the late 1960s in an attempt to "cool out" the Black Panther Party and other radical Black organizations.[22] It has continued into the 1980s, as CIA shipments of cocaine have been used not only to fund the anti-Nicaraguan contras, but also to quell domestic unrest.[23]

Continuing economic exploitation of people of color is another key aspect of institutional racism. As in the case of white women, there have been some significant changes in the economic status of people of color in the past three decades. Yet, at the same time that *employed* Black men have been making higher wages, a smaller and smaller proportion of all Black men have been able to find jobs at all.[24] While Black women have experienced gains in terms of employment and income, they have increasingly gained sole financial responsibility for their children. This is, of course, related to the fact that more Black men are unable to find jobs, and are therefore unable to contribute to family income. As of 1985, over 44 percent of Black families with children were maintained by women.[25] As a result of this combined racism and sexism, *more than half the African-American children in this country are currently being raised in poverty.*[26] The implications for these women and their children, in terms of receiving quality health care for AIDS, are devastating.

Racist imagery in educational materials and the media continues to indicate the institutional nature of U.S. racism. Crimes that victimize people of color often are not deemed "newsworthy" (whereas crimes with white victims are). Events that primarily or disproportionately affect communities of color (such as the AIDS epidemic) are not thought to be of interest to the "general reader," who is assumed to be white and usually male. The illness and deaths of people of color, women, and lesbians and gay men are simply not deemed to be "important" enough to report.

Class Oppression and AIDS

In addition to the issue of unequal access to treatment, this country's response to the AIDS crisis in general is profoundly influenced by its class structure and its profit-driven economy. For example, treatments that will not be profitable simply are not explored by major drug companies and are undertaken rarely by the government. Personal and financial connections between major pharmaceutical companies and the government agencies responsible for regulating these companies' AIDS research programs further complicate the problem.

This is particularly important in the case of women, intravenous drug users (IVDUs), and others with lower incomes. A drug company can't make a profit on a drug if many of the people who need it are too poor to pay a high price for it. Research and drug trials tend to be concentrated among those people with enough money to make an experimental drug "profitable."

Attention to profitability, rather than to saving lives, also leads to "turf wars" and patent battles that further delay experimental drugs and even proven treatments from reaching patients who need them. For example, in 1986, Michael McGrath of the University of California at San Francisco found that trichosanthin ("Compound Q") killed HIV-infected immune system cells in the test tube. However, he waited two years to announce his discovery, until he and his pharmaceutical sponsor, Genelabs, could obtain a patent on the product and sell its licensing rights worldwide. Compound Q may or may not prove to be an effective treatment for AIDS, but the research on this vital question was delayed for two years for purely financial gain.[27]

Heterosexism and AIDS

As with sexism, heterosexism refers not just to the attitudes of individuals. Rather, a pressure towards heterosexuality is built into most of our major social, economic, and political institutions.

Violence against lesbians, bisexuals, and gay men is often tolerated and/or initiated by police. A recent survey showed that 90 percent of lesbians and gay men interviewed had experienced heterosexist violence, or the threat of such violence, during their lifetimes.[28]

Lesbians, gay men, and bisexuals suffer from institutional forms of economic discrimination in addition to direct housing and job discrimination. Gay men and lesbians lack spousal health care benefits for ourselves and our children, marital tax breaks, "family" status in rental agreements, the legal right to make decisions for our lovers in emergencies (including medical emergencies), and even inheritance rights in the case of the death of a lover.

As discussed earlier, lesbians and gay men are frequently denied reproductive rights, including alternative insemination for lesbians, adoption and foster care, and child custody rights in contested cases.

The heterosexist imagery and ideas put forth in the mass media and by religious and educational institutions, among others, perpetuate the notion that heterosexuality is the only "natural" or "moral" sexuality. The authorities of many major religions also state or strongly imply that homophobia and heterosexism are acceptable, even divinely sanctioned. Some even claim that AIDS is God's "punishment" for sexual or other behaviors that they consider to be unacceptable. This propaganda has a major impact on federal, state, and local governments' AIDS policies and funding.

Ableism and AIDS

Ableism consists of the practices, behaviors, and attitudes that deny disabled people, including people with AIDS (PWAs), access to all or most of the major institutions of this society. One in six Americans is disabled,[29] but our visibility, earning ability, and political clout are far smaller than our numbers. Violence against the disabled happens throughout our society, yet the media totally overlook the existence of such violence. Visibly disabled women are often perceived to be "easy prey," and are significantly more likely to be assaulted than able-bodied women.[30] In addition, violence against PWAs (or those who are *believed* to have AIDS) is on the rise in most urban communities.[31]

Economic and insurance discrimination is another major aspect of institutional ableism. The incomes of employed disabled people are significantly lower than those of the able-bodied; disabled women earn only 36 percent of what nondisabled men make.[32] Direct employment discrimination against the disabled is often compounded by inaccessibility and discrimination on the part of schools and universities. Despite the existence of Section 504 of the Rehabilitation Act (which mandates appropriate education for all children, regardless of ability level), many disabled children still do not receive the special education they need to become economically self-sufficient adults.

In addition to lower income, disabled people often have higher medical costs than the able-bodied, and are, ironically, much less able to get health insurance. It is perfectly legal for insurance companies to deny policies to those with HIV illness, or other "preexisting medical conditions," and to refuse to pay benefits if people conceal their disabilities to get insurance. The combination of lower incomes, higher medical costs, and lack of insurance often results in very low standards of living for the disabled, especially disabled women and disabled people of color.

Ableism also perpetuates discrimination in the accessibility of buildings and transportation. This society was literally not built for the disabled. The vast majority of streets and sidewalks, apartment buildings, stores, and offices are totally inaccessible to wheelchair users. Until recently, federal law did not require chair lifts on publicly funded buses, drastically limiting many disabled people's mobility. In public facilities it is still unusual to find hearing interpretation or Braille, which would greatly increase mobility and autonomy for the hearing- and sight-impaired.

Disabled people are often denied control over their reproductive capability. In the early 1900s, as a result of the eugenics movement and Social Darwinism, most states had laws on the books requiring sterilization for the physically disabled, epileptics, and the "feebleminded." Although by and large these laws are no longer enforced, involuntary sterilization of the disabled continues, especially among the developmentally disabled and disabled people of color.[33]

Despite being supposedly "nondirective," many genetic counselors continue to "direct" women with genetically passed disabilities to seriously consider sterilization or abortion. Pregnant HIV-positive women are often coerced into abortions, despite the fact that only 20 to 50 percent of their children will actually receive the virus. Even some feminists defend abortion on the grounds that women must have the right to abort "defective" fetuses, including those that have a chance of being HIV positive. These arguments assume that no woman would choose to give birth to a disabled fetus, and that disability is a "personal tragedy," rather than a political and social problem of accessibility and funding for services and health care.

Rarely, if ever, are PWAs and other disabled people portrayed as normal and productive members of society. When we're not totally invisible, disabled people are usually portrayed in the media as pitiful, childlike victims. We're portrayed as asexual and unable to carry on personal or romantic relationships, whether heterosexual or lesbian or gay.

The media and the medical profession share the notion that disability is something to be overcome, that we must "strive to overcome our disabilities" rather than learn to live within our capabilities. The underlying assumption, of course, is that there is something terribly wrong with the disabled person, rather than with the social structure in which she or he lives.

All these types of oppression reduce women's access to the information, resources, and political clout necessary to fight AIDS. Women in general enter the AIDS crisis from a more vulnerable position than do men. Women who face additional forms of oppression are that much more vulnerable. Solving the AIDS crisis for *everyone* means combating the powerlessness and marginalization of many of the oppressed people in this country: women, people of color, the poor, and the disabled. As AIDS activists, we have a responsibility to plan our actions in ways that take account of the differences among women, as well as our similarities. The information in the rest of this book will help us all to do that.

Notes

1. Federal Bureau of Investigation, *Uniform Crime Report: Crime in the United States*, 1980, p. 15. The FBI adds the following footnote to their statistical estimate: "Even with the advent of rape crisis centers and the improved awareness by police dealing with rape victims, forcible rape, a violent crime against a person, is still recognized as one of the most under-reported of all Index crimes...Victims' fear of their assailants' return and their embarrassment over the incidents are just two factors which can override their decision to contact law enforcement."
2. Audre Lorde, "An Open Letter to Mary Daly," in *This Bridge Called My Back: Writings by Radical Women of Color*, Cherríe Moraga and Gloria Anzaldúa, eds. (Albany, NY: Kitchen Table: Women of Color Press, 1983), p. 97.
3. *Uniform Crime Report*, p. 15.
4. Lenore Walker, *The Battered Woman* (New York: Harper and Row, 1979), p. 14.
5. Ronnie Sandroff, "Sexual Harassment in the Fortune 500," in *Working Woman*, December 1988, pp. 69-73.
6. Sources for varying estimates:
   - Susan Forward and Craig Buck, *The Betrayal of Innocence: Incest and Its Devastation* (New York: Penguin, 1978), p. 3.
   - Judith Herman and Lisa Hirschman, "Father-Daughter Incest," in *Signs: A Journal of Women and Culture*, Vol. 2, no. 4, Summer 1977, pp. 735-756.
   - Kee MacFarlane, "The Sexual Abuse of Children," in Jane Chapman and Margaret Gates, eds., *The Victimization of Women* (Beverly Hills, CA: Sage Publications, 1978), pp. 81-109.
7. *Economic Report of the President*, 1989, Table B-37.
8. Derived from "Money Income of Households, Families and Persons in the United States: 1986," U.S. Department of Commerce, Bureau of the Census.
9. "Money Income of Households..." Bureau of the Census.
10. "Divorces and Annulments, Rate and Percent Distribution, by Sex and Age, 1985," in *Statistical Abstract of the United States, 1989* (U.S. Department of Commerce, Bureau of the Census), p. 87.
11. Ruth Sidel, *Women and Children Last* (New York: Penguin, 1986), p. 18.
12. Nancy Folbre, *Field Guide to the U.S. Economy* (New York: Pantheon Books, 1987), Graphs 3-11.
13. Folbre, *Field Guide*.
14. John Bohne, Tom Cunningham, Jon Engbretson, Ken Fornataro, and Mark Harrington, *T+D Handbook: Treatment Decisions*, ACT UP/New York, unpublished, 1989, p. 32.
15. Joseph Pleck, *Working Wives, Working Husbands* (Beverly Hills, CA:

Sage Publications, 1985).

16. Pleck, *Working Wives,* p. 121.
17. Pleck, *Working Wives,* p. 123.
18. Arlie Hochschild, *The Second Shift: Working Parents and the Revolution at Home* (New York: Viking, 1989), p. 4.
19. Susan Davis and CARASA (Committee for Abortion Rights and Against Sterilization Abuse), *Women Under Attack: Victories, Backlash, and the Fight for Reproductive Freedom* (Boston: South End Press, 1988), p. 22.
20. Ann Northrop, Hetrick Martin Institute, personal communication.
21. William Brennan, Dissenting Opinion in *McClesky v. Kemp,* U.S. Supreme Court Reporter, Vol. 107, 1987, pp. 1756-1794.
22. Leslie Cockburn, *Out of Control* (New York: Viking, 1988).
23. Cockburn, *Out of Control.*
24. Kimberly Christensen, "Political Determinants of Income Changes for African-American Women and Men," submitted for publication to *Review of Radical Political Economics* in June 1990.
25. Folbre, *Field Guide.*
26. Sidel, *Women and Children Last,* p. 3.
27. Bohne et al., *T+D Handbook: Treatment Decisions,* p. 44.
28. Survey conducted by National Gay and Lesbian Task Force, New York, 1988.
29. Barbara Mandell Altman, "Disabled Women and the Social Structure," in *With the Power of Each Breath: A Disabled Women's Anthology,* Susan Browne, Debra Conners, and Nanci Stern, eds. (San Francisco: Cleis Press, 1985), pp. 69-76.
30. Rebecca Grothaus, "Abuse of Women with Disabilities," in *With the Power of Each Breath,* pp. 124-128.
31. Survey conducted by the National Gay and Lesbian Task Force, New York, 1988.
32. Altman, "Disabled Women and the Social Structure."
33. Anne Finger, "Reproductive Rights and Disability," in *With the Power of Each Breath,* pp. 292-307.

Transmission Issues for Women

CYNTHIA CHRIS

Obstacles to Safer Sex: Am I at Risk?

AIDS is thought to be caused by a virus called HIV which is transmitted when the blood, menstrual fluid, semen, or vaginal secretions of an infected person enter another person's body by unsafe sex, unsafe needle use, unscreened transfusions of blood or blood products, or from mother to fetus through the placenta. Many women—and men—believe they are not at risk and do not need to practice safe sex or change needle-sharing habits. To assess your own risk for contracting HIV, answer the following yes-or-no questions for the years 1977 to the present:

- Have you used drugs or alcohol to the point of impaired judgment and memory loss, so that you went home with someone and don't remember what you did?
- Have you had unsafe sex (see "Safer Sex" section below) by consent or by force?
- Did you receive a blood transfusion or blood products before 1985? (In mid-1985 a test was developed to screen blood for HIV; later transfusions pose virtually no risk.)
- Have you shared unsterilized hypodermic needles or other drug works, or shared unsterilized needles for tattooing or piercing the skin?
- Have you had a needlestick injury involving an HIV-positive blood sample?
- Have you had unscreened alternative insemination?
- Have you had unsafe sex involving oral or manual contact with blood or vaginal fluids of a woman who has shared unsterilized drug works, or who has had unsafe sex with a man?

If you answered yes to any of these questions, you may be at risk for HIV infection.[1] Of course, the accuracy of any risk assessment depends on your honesty and the honesty of your partner.

Ours is a sex-negative and woman-negative society. Sex is frequently seen as something dangerous, dirty, and not to be discussed. For women, sex that is not specifically for procreation is often associated with unwanted pregnancies, sexually transmitted diseases (STDs), and harsh moral judgments, while the pleasures of sex are mainly reserved for men, on whom society does not impose such strict standards regarding sex before or outside of marriage. Fear of AIDS has increased many people's fear of sex, and many of us—women and men, straight, bisexual, lesbian, and gay—have a difficult time talking about our sexual histories and sexual practices with our partners. We may fear that safe sex practices will reduce our pleasure or the pleasure of our lovers, or that our lovers will leave us if we insist on safer sex. But with education about how HIV is transmitted and how to protect ourselves and our partners from it, we know that we can have sex that is both safe and pleasurable.

Yet safety and pleasure are concepts that many women tend not to associate with sex. Society teaches women not to like our bodies, not to know anything about them, and not to touch ourselves. We are taught that the pleasure of our partners (who are assumed to be male) comes before our own pleasure, that our orgasms are not as important as theirs. Likewise, birth control is almost always regarded as the woman's responsibility. A man who is reluctant to use condoms for contraception or to prevent STDs may also be unwilling to use condoms to prevent the transmission of HIV. He may be reluctant to use condoms, believing that only gay men get AIDS, that he can't get AIDS if he doesn't do drugs, or that condom use is against his religion. A woman may not insist on condoms if she fears that the man may beat her up, that he will leave her for someone who won't make him use condoms, or that she will get paid more or get more drugs if she doesn't make him use a condom.

Properly used, condoms protect against the transmission of HIV and STDs, as well as unwanted pregnancy, but no other form of birth control protects you or your partner from HIV, including the pill, IUD, diaphragm, cervical cap, sponge, sterilization, rhythm method, or *coitus interruptus* (withdrawal). The use of condoms must become an integral part of sex education. Parents must teach their children about safer sex and contraception, and each of us must advocate for safer-sex information and practices within our peer groups.

Among lesbians, cases of AIDS have been largely uncounted and vastly underpublicized.[2] Those of us who are lesbians may believe that we are not at risk, or that lesbian sex is safe, so "safer" sex is unnecessary. We may assume that all lesbians are HIV negative. We deny that we may have put ourselves at risk, although many of us have used IV drugs, many of us had unprotected sex with men in the past, many of us continue to have sex with men although we continue to identify ourselves as lesbians, and many of us have had unprotected oral sex with a woman partner who may have been exposed to the virus. As well, lack of safe-sex information addressed to lesbians, and unfamiliarity with and difficulty in finding dental dams, discourage us from seeing ourselves as at risk and from practicing safer sex.

Safer Sex

Safer sex is a way of taking control of, and taking responsibility for, one's sexual behavior. It allows us to protect ourselves and our partners against the transmission of HIV. As well, safer sex, practiced consistently and correctly, can protect us against unwanted pregnancies and STDs such as syphilis, gonorrhea, chlamydia, chancroid, herpes, and hepatitis B. Safer sex protects people who are HIV positive from reinfection with the virus, which can accelerate suppression of the immune system, and from other infections that may have little effect on a healthy immune system but could be devastating if one's immunity is compromised. Safer-sex practices recognize that sex is not only intercourse between a woman's vagina and a man's penis. Sex can involve any part of the body. It may be heterosexual, gay, or lesbian, and it may take place in monogamous relationships or among a number of partners.

The challenge of safer sex is for partners to allow for as much and as varied stimulation as they desire without putting each other at risk. In order to determine what safer sex is, as well as what is risky or unsafe, it is important to remember that while arousal—the physical responses to direct or indirect stimulation of the clitoris, which may lead to orgasm—is basically the same for all women; what *causes* arousal varies from woman to woman.

Safe sex includes masturbation, exhibitionism (showing off), voyeurism (watching someone else), fantasy, talking, massage, rubbing bodies together (humping, sometimes known among lesbians as tribadism or by the French word *frottage*), and other safe activities that do not allow blood, semen, or vaginal secretions to be exchanged among partners.

As well, safe sex can include penetration of a woman's vagina (cunt, pussy) or anus (asshole) by her partner's fingers or penis (cock, dick), or by a dildo. She may enjoy oral sex; "going down" on one's partner may consist of mouth-to-vulva contact (cunnilingus, eating pussy), mouth-to-penis contact (fellatio, giving head), or mouth-to-anus contact (anilingus, rimming). A woman may do water sports or scat, sexual activities involving urine or feces (piss or shit). She may participate in S & M (sadomasochism) or B & D (bondage and discipline). All of these activities can be performed safely, so that blood, semen, and vaginal fluids do not enter your or your partner's bloodstream through the mouth, vagina, anus, cuts, or other openings in the skin.

Barriers are the best protection currently available. They include latex condoms (rubbers), dental dams (square sheets of latex used by dentists and now recommended for oral sex), heavy-gauge household plastic wrap, latex surgical gloves, and fingercots, which fit over one finger instead of the whole hand. With latex barriers, a water-based lubricant such as K-Y or H-R Jelly must be used. Do not use oil- or petroleum-based lubes such as Vaseline, vegetable oils, moisturizing lotions, or mineral oil; they dissolve latex and make it break. It's best to choose lubes like Forplay or Astroglide, which are water based and may contain nonoxynol-9 or octoxynol-9, so-called spermicides that decrease the movement of sperm and therefore its ability to cause pregnancy; they also inhibit the transmission of HIV. Contraceptive foams and gels made for use with diaphragms (PrePair, Conceptrol, Ramses) contain nonoxynol-9 and make effective lubes. However, these spermicides may cause allergic reactions or skin or vaginal irritations. They may also disrupt vaginal organisms that help ward off some types of opportunistic infections.

Blood and semen contain the highest concentration of HIV. Vaginal secretions have a lower concentration of HIV, but high enough to create a risk of transmission (this remains controversial enough to warrant further discussion below). Although HIV is found in trace amounts in saliva, sweat, and tears, there is no evidence that HIV can be transmitted through these fluids.

Medical journals have documented the transmission of HIV to one heterosexual man and at least six lesbians who contracted HIV by going down on an infected woman.[3] (Because saliva does not contain enough HIV to transmit the virus, the possibility of transmission from an infected person to someone he or she is eating out is extremely low, but bleeding or infections in the mouth and cuts or genital sores such as those caused by some STDs could make the risk viable.)

The risk posed by vaginal secretions alone is relatively low, but it can be raised easily by several factors. The amount of fluids produced during sex varies, and some women have a copious ejaculation of fluid when they orgasm (come). If a woman is HIV infected and has a lot of vaginal secretions, the amount of HIV to which her partner is exposed during unprotected oral sex is increased. Also, many women have traces of vaginal infections, such as chlamydia or yeast. Vaginal discharges resulting from infections contain white blood cells, which contain HIV and therefore increase the concentration of HIV in vaginal fluids.

Any amount of blood, even one so small that it is imperceptible, can contain enough HIV to cause infection. Up to three days before or after a woman's period there may be blood you can't see in her secretions. Vigorous fucking of any kind can abrade the vaginal walls and cause bleeding you may not be aware of.

Get to know what a healthy vagina and labia look like. By looking at your vagina with a mirror, a plastic speculum, and a flashlight; by having your partner look at your labia; or by looking at your partner's vagina with the lights on before you have oral sex, you can identify infections and other conditions such as sores, bleeding, or cuts that may increase your risk of being exposed to or transmitting HIV.

For the person doing the licking or sucking, susceptibility to HIV is influenced by how healthy he or she is from lips to stomach. For example, cold sores, bleeding gums, sore throats, and ulcers are openings that would permit HIV to enter a person's bloodstream. Even if you have no obvious cuts or sores, you may want to avoid brushing or flossing your teeth, which can cause bleeding, and smoking, which can open up blood vessels in your throat, just before or after oral sex.

During vaginal or anal intercourse, use a latex condom and a water-based lubricant, preferably one containing nonoxynol-9 (this applies both to heterosexuals and to men who have anal sex with other men). Unwrap the condom carefully so that it does not tear. Put a drop of lube inside the tip of the rubber, and unroll it down the shaft of the penis all the way to its base. Some condoms have reservoirs at the tip for the cum; if it doesn't, hold onto a half-inch at the tip while you unroll it. Put some lube on the outside of the rubber, as well as on the vagina or anus. Unlike your vagina, your asshole does not lubricate itself during sex, so use extra lube to help prevent the rubber from breaking. You can "double-bag" (use two condoms at once), but put lube inside only the first one; if you put lube in between rubbers, they may slip off. After sex, remove the condom carefully so that no semen spills out. Never re-use a condom, and always use latex condoms—lambskin is porous and does not provide adequate protection against HIV.[4]

For performing oral sex on a man, he should wear a condom from start to finish. Use unlubed condoms—prelubed condoms taste bad. You can make a "head condom" by fitting the rubber over only the tip of the penis rather than all the way down the shaft. Pre-cum (fluid that seeps out of the penis before ejaculation), like semen, poses a risk of HIV transmission. If you are healthy from your lips to your stomach (see above), risk of exposure to HIV may be reduced during a blow job without protection, if you don't let your partner ejaculate in your mouth, or if you don't swallow his cum.

A condom can also be used on a dildo. If you put a sex toy into the vagina, put a new condom on it before you put it into the anus, and vice versa. Likewise, put a new condom on it before sharing the toy with your partner. If they are shared without condoms, dildos and vibrators should be washed with a solution of ten parts water to one part bleach and rinsed well between uses.

Cunnilingus is safe when a barrier is used to cover the vagina. As yet the most common barrier, dental dams are six-by-six-inch latex squares, often flavored with chocolate or mint. New dams are coated with talc and should be rinsed with water and dried before using; a water-based lube, preferably with nonoxynol-9, should be applied to the side that will touch the vagina. Don't share and don't re-use dams. Dental dams are not widely available—medical supply houses or gay and lesbian health organizations may be the best sources. You may find dams difficult to hold in place; one solution is to sew them into crotchless panties.

A latex barrier that has not yet been tested by many safe sex advocates is called Thera-band. Produced in six-inch-wide rolls for physical therapists, it comes in a variety of thicknesses. A six-yard roll should cost approximately $10 from a medical supply outlet. You can also cut the tips off condoms and slit the remaining piece lengthwise to make a flat square which is thinner but narrower than a dam, making it even trickier to hold in place. Doing similar surgery on latex gloves results in a latex patch that is thinner than a dental dam and larger than a slit condom.

Another alternative to dental dams is ordinary plastic wrap (Saran, Handi-Wrap, etc.), which is untested but recommended by many safer-sex educators. It's easy to get and you can tear off a piece which is large enough to hold easily, but not all brands are heavy enough; to test for porousness, wrap a cut onion in the plastic—if you can still smell it, it is not thick enough to prevent HIV from passing through.

For rimming, use a dental dam (or a substitute) with a water-based, spermicidal lube. Unprotected rimming is considered unsafe because microscopic fecal matter that gets into your mouth may contain blood as well as bacteria that can cause other infections. If you've used a dam on the vagina, use another one on the anus.

Latex gloves and fingercots are recommended for anal and vaginal finger-fucking and fisting if you have cuts on your hands or openings caused by biting or clipping your nails too short, and if there may be blood, fecal matter, or discharges caused by infections in your partner's vagina or anus. Look at your hands before you put them inside someone. A bit of lube inside the glove improves its sensitivity.[5]

Safer Needle Use

If you share needles with another person for any reason—to inject drugs, to pierce ears or other parts of the body, or for tattooing—his or her blood enters your bloodstream, and you risk infection with HIV, hepatitis, or other blood-borne infections. It does not matter what kinds of drugs are being injected—narcotics, cocaine, speed, steroids, or prescription drugs—and it does not matter if you skin pop or shoot directly into the veins.

If you use intravenous drugs, get your own needles and works; don't use anyone else's needles or other equipment; don't share any part of your works, including needles, syringes, and cookers; and don't share or re-use cottons. If you have to share, or if you rent works at a shooting gallery, clean them thoroughly before you use them. Don't use rebagged needles; they may look sterile but probably aren't.

Clean your works (or needles being used for tattooing or piercing) with rubbing alcohol or a solution of ten parts water and one part household bleach (Clorox). Draw the alcohol or bleach solution into the syringe through the needles and squirt it out at least three times; then take the works apart and soak them for ten minutes. Rinse everything thoroughly in running water.

Needles which you may encounter when you are being treated in a hospital or by a doctor, dentist, or acupuncturist are either disposable (meaning they are only used once and then thrown away) or they are sterilized between uses, eliminating any risk of infection. Donating blood poses no risk, and receiving transfusions of blood and blood products has been virtually risk free since the HIV-antibody test was developed in 1985.

Resources

More information about safer-sex and needle sharing is available from a number of AIDS and health organizations. Some have telephone hotlines, and many have published pamphlets. Read these with a critical eye, as the quality of these materials varies greatly. Consider the following excerpt:

> It is not the number of previous lovers you or your partner have had but the amount of unprotected sex either of you have had. Consistent safer-sex with a number of partners may be less risky than unprotected sex with just one partner if that person is infected.[6]

Contrast this with an excerpt from a pamphlet by the American College of Obstetricians-Gynecologists:

> Limit your partners...the safest kind of sexual relationship is one that is mutually monogamous. If either you or your partner has sex with other people keep in mind that with each sex partner, the chance of getting infected rises.

The first excerpt is sex positive, takes into account that the reality of many women's lives is not permanent mutual monogamy, and offers safe sex as a viable choice. The second reinforces fear of sex and offers advice that many women are not able or willing to follow. We can't simply demand safer-sex information. We must be aware that the kind of safer-sex information and materials that women need are those which are relevant to our cultures and our lives.

Notes

1. This risk assessment survey is modeled after those used by safe-sex educators, including Denise Ribble, R.N., and Diane Jeep Reis. See Ribble, "Not Just Another Article on Lesbian Safe Sex," *Sappho's Isle,* July 1989, p. 15.
2. Early in 1989, the CDC counted 164 AIDS cases among self-identified lesbians and bisexual women. See Lena Einhorn, "New Data on Lesbians and AIDS," *off our backs,* April 1989, p. 10. More recently, CDC officials have reported in personal communications that the data have been "cleaned up" and that there are only 100 cases of AIDS among women who have reported having sex with other women.
3. See Donna Minkowitz, "Safe and Sappho: An AIDS Primer for Lesbians," *The Village Voice,* February 21, 1989, p. 21.
4. See also "The Safer Sex Condom Guide for Men and Women" (New York: Gay Men's Health Crisis, 1987). Available from GMHC, 129 W. 20th St., New York, NY 10011, (212) 807-6655.
5. For more information on risk assessment, transmission, and safe sex, see Cindy Patton and Janis Kelly, *Making It: A Woman's Guide to Sex in the Age of AIDS/Haciéndolo: Guía para Mujeres en la Era del SIDA* (Ithaca,

NY: Firebrand Books, 1987, revised and updated 1988).
6. "Women & AIDS" (Rockville, MD: American College Health Association, 1988). Available from ACHA, 15879 Crabbs Branch Way, Rockville, MD 20855, (301) 963-1100. For more information on safer sex and needle use, consult the resources at the end of this book.

Safe Sex Is Real Sex

ZOE LEONARD

I have a lover who is HIV positive.

I am HIV negative.

I want to talk about my experience with safe sex and loving someone who is HIV positive.

Safe sex is often spoken about as a major drag...necessary, but fundamentally unerotic. People never seem to say, "Yeah, I do this with my lover and it's really hot."

Well, I do it with my lover and it's really hot.

I knew he was HIV positive before I slept with him. I had felt surprised when I found out; he just looked so damned healthy. I didn't envision having a sexual relationship with him, mainly because I've been an out and happy lesbian for years. So, when we realized we had crushes on each other, it was a big shock and really scary. I was doing AIDS activism and supposedly I knew all about safe sex, but suddenly I couldn't remember what I knew. All the grey areas of "low-risk" and "safer" sex seemed unclear and menacing; was kissing really OK? Secret fears snuck in. What if everyone is wrong about safe sex, about saliva? I felt I couldn't ask about these scary thoughts, like I should know the answers and had no right to feel so threatened. I didn't want to reinforce the stigma that he fights: feeling infectious, reading about himself as an "AIDS carrier." It had been relatively easy to be supportive and accepting of my friends with AIDS, to be sex positive, to talk about safe sex, but now it was in my bedroom, and I'm wondering: can he put his finger inside me without a glove, can he go down on me, can I touch his penis? Safe sex is different when you know your partner is infected. I don't want to appear frightened. I don't want to make him feel bad by talking about it, but I really, really don't want to get infected. (I tested negative for HIV about two years ago, and swore that I would never again place myself at any risk whatsoever.) And, here I was, a dyke at that, kissing this man good-night after our first date.

In the beginning I was overwhelmed, terrified after that first kiss. So, we didn't dive right into bed and "do the nasty." We took our time and messed around for months, figuring out what we were comfortable with. It was great, all that sex building up. I always came, but we never did anything outside the strictest confines of "no risk" sex without talking about it first. We talked a lot about limits and seeing each other's points of view: my understanding that he doesn't want to feel like a pariah, or like he represents disease, his understanding that I had a right to be frightened, cautious, curious. It is important that I never do anything out of pressure, out of a need to prove that I'm not prejudiced. I realize that, as much as he cares about my health, I have to decide for myself what is safe, and stick to it. I knew I would resent him if we did something I wasn't sure about, and I would fly into a panic the next day.

I also realize that he is at risk for any infection that I might be carrying, and that safe sex is to protect him, too. A mild infection that might be harmless to me could be devastating to him.

I'm afraid of making him sick. I had hepatitis this summer, and we were worried that I might give it to him. Hepatitis can be very dangerous to anyone with an impaired immune system. I felt frightened and guilty. Later on I got angry that my *being* sick was somewhat overlooked in the panic surrounding the possibility of his *getting* sick. I found myself anxious and worried about his health at a time when I needed comfort and care. Sometimes I don't feel legitimate in feeling sorry for myself or being concerned about my own health.

A great thing about safe sex is that we aren't "fuck-o-centric." We don't have intercourse all the time. We get off a lot of different ways, so our sex is varied and we don't just fall into one pattern.

The main thing is not to form a hierarchy of what "real sex" is, or equate "real sex" with high-risk practices. We can't think that humping is fake and intercourse is real.

Condoms are great. They are really sexy to me now, like lingerie or the perfume of a lover. Maybe I'm just immature, or particularly responsive to Pavlovian training, but the mere sight of condoms, lube, or dental dams sends a sexy feeling through me. The tools of safe sex become as significant and fetishized as other toys for pleasure. I'm always hearing about how condoms and other latex barriers take away all the spontaneity, as if sex before AIDS was always spontaneous and perfect. There are many barriers to good sex, like being too anxious, too busy, or too tired, or the *phone ringing,* or not finding someone you want to have sex with in the first place.

You can use safe sex to tease each other, waiting until you want something really badly before you screw up the courage to ask for it (or beg for it). Then you stop, and hang in this state of anticipation, feeling like a teenager, waiting while he (for instance) gets the first condom out, squirts the lube in it, and gets it on. Then he gets the second condom out and on. It's tense and full of anticipation, and I rarely feel either of us cooling off. It can be exciting to admit what you want, to articulate it, and to know what your partner wants, and to use the confines of safe sex to create tension and escalate desire.

Also, it can be a gift, like the time we went away for the weekend and he showed up with a shopping bag full of every form of latex known to humankind. It's a way of showing that you care about someone's health, and that you want him or her to be considerate and romantic at the same time.

We've had to negotiate so many aspects of our relationship that otherwise might have remained mute, but this has given us the context to discuss other things: what feels good, what we want, what freaks us out. The need to figure all those things out has built trust between us; it's made us honest.

But divisions do occur between the sick and the well. My lover is asymptomatic, so HIV often seems like an abstract issue to me. When I'm talking about something in the future, he blurts out, "I don't know if I'll be alive in five years." Can I understand the depression? I feel guilty sometimes and cut off other times.

It's one thing to learn to fuck safely and quite another to feel committed to someone that you are afraid might get really sick or die. I think: can I do it? Will I have the patience, will I be adequate? What if he really does get sick, what then?...can I handle feeling this responsible? Do I want to take care of him? And what if he really does die? What about that?

I've had friends die of AIDS. I have visceral memories of Dan in the hospital just before he died, massaging his feet, feeling the thick lumps of KS lesions through his sweat socks. I remember him semi-conscious, making noises, responding to the pressure of my hands, his lover saying yes, he likes that.

I was once very much in love with a woman who got cancer. For a year my whole world telescoped into just her room, her health. My life was filled with nightmares and worrying, cooking, obsessing. My days were spent in the hospital, knowing the staff, being a regular. I knew every detail of her treatment, read all the articles, took notes. Running into friends, everyone would ask, "How's Simone?" People stopped asking, "How are you?" There was a certain relief in turning myself over to this greater cause, where everything was always about her—humidifiers, macrobiotic food, appointments. Even now, we are friends, and still there is a subtext: will she get sick again, will she die?

I wonder, do I just thrive on drama? Do I have a martyr complex, or a death wish? Did I fall for him because of his status? Do I want to get infected; is this my most recent and subtle form of self-destruction? Friends and family are anxious, ask me about *it*. They tell me I'm crazy, and speak of illness and health in hushed tones.

And I have to admit, after all these months, sometimes I'm still scared. I see an article and I think, could I be the first case of saliva transmission? Why am I still scared? I forget for weeks, and then when I get sick, feverish, peaked, HIV is there like a threat. I worry secretly, and when I tell him, he's angry, defensive.

All around us, his friends, my friends, into the hospital, out of the hospital, dying. When will it start with him? He gets a cold, the flu. He's tired, glands swollen.

I hate this virus.

This started out to be about the joys of safe sex, but I guess it's complicated.

I am HIV negative, as of my last test. I've learned a lot and had some really hot sex and lots of flirty, sexy stuff, and there's been a lot of love and happiness in this relationship. There's a difference between rational fears and irrational ones. I try to act on the rational ones. I try to protect myself and my lover from real threats, and try to overcome the irrational fears.

You *can* make decisions about your life and love based on what you want, and not let illness, or fear of illness, make all the decisions for you.

Unique Aspects of HIV Infection in Women

RISA DENENBERG

What Is Not Known

A woman with HIV illness who lives in Newark, New Jersey, lives an average of 15.5 weeks following a diagnosis of AIDS,[1] while a white gay male in the northeast region of the United States with HIV illness lives an average of 20.8 months following diagnosis.[2] There are many problems in assessing the number of women with AIDS, as well as the ways in which HIV disease affects women.

Very little is known about women and HIV disease, and very little research has been done or can be anticipated. Therefore, it is not possible to draw conclusions about risk factors, disease progression, opportunistic infections, or proper treatments. However, by framing the relevant questions, we can provide a basis for understanding what we need to know.

In this discussion it is important to remember that women's bodies are different from men's in significant ways, that women are rarely viewed as individuals in the health care system and often are viewed as vectors for disease, and that women rarely see primary health care practitioners and often receive health care in settings where public health concerns have more priority than individual concerns. Additionally, women delay seeking care due to, for example, a lack of resources, the burden of child care and caring for elderly or ill family members, our being lesbians and afraid of discrimination, or the fact that so often our complaints of fatigue, headaches, and weight loss are assumed by ourselves and others to be "merely" emotional or stress related.

If we want to understand what happens to a woman after exposure to HIV, women activists will have to be willing to ask publicly the relevant questions.

Why Do Women Die Faster than Men?

Approximately 73 percent of women with AIDS in the United States are women of color, yet people of color comprise only approximately 25 percent of the overall population. Of women diagnosed with AIDS, 52 percent are Black, 27 percent are white, 20 percent are Latina, 0.6 percent are Asian/Pacific Islander, and 0.2 percent are Native American. Women constitute nearly 9 percent of the total number of AIDS cases in the United States reported to the Centers for Disease Control (CDC) through December 1989. Forty percent of men with AIDS are men of color.[3] The disproportionate representation of people of color of both sexes, but especially of women of color, reflects the unique social and economic burdens encountered in living in the United States, and also explains, in part, the mortality differences between all women and white men. For example, a Black woman intravenous drug user (IVDU) with pneumocystis carinii pneumonia (PCP) has the least favorable survival time of any group of AIDS patients studied.

Statistics on women and mortality also reflect the reality that women as a group are undercounted, overlooked, misdiagnosed, and undiagnosed. Further, women are generally treated inadequately following a diagnosis.

This occurs in the following ways.

- Diagnosis comes late in the course of a woman's illness. This occurs because women do not have access to health care or because they delay health care due to other priorities such as finding housing and feeding children. It also occurs because most health care providers are inadequately trained to identify HIV disease and don't even look for it in women. Women with HIV often die soon after they are diagnosed; often diagnoses of HIV are not made until after their deaths.

- Women are underdiagnosed. The CDC has specific guidelines for what constitutes a diagnosis of AIDS. They were last updated in 1987, and many new cases are currently being identified on the basis of that revision. Still, both the initial and the updated guidelines show that AIDS is primarily understood as a white gay men's disease. Women simply do not fit into this disease pattern. Therefore, women often die with AIDS-related complex (ARC), which is generally understood as a stepping stone from asymptomatic illness to AIDS and is usually diagnosed when someone demonstrates HIV-related symptoms such as weight loss, swollen glands, and fever, but does not meet the CDC's definition of AIDS. Since many women die of ARC (the numbers are unknown because deaths from ARC are not tracked as are deaths from AIDS), it is logical to assume that the CDC guidelines are inadequate for diagnosing AIDS in women; without adequate diagnoses, the quality of treatment offered to women is undoubtedly compromised. Equally serious for these women is the fact that, without AIDS diagnoses, they do not qualify for particular benefits available only to people with AIDS.

- Women are misdiagnosed. They often die of HIV-related illnesses that are not recognized as such. Perhaps less time and money are spent on diagnostic tests or on discovering the causes of a woman's symptoms. Again, women are not viewed by health care providers as being likely to have HIV disease. For example, between 1981 and 1988, there was an unexplained and significant increase of deaths from pneumonia and influenza in women aged 15 to 44 in several urban centers in the United States.[4] Many of these deaths might have been from undiagnosed opportunistic infections common to HIV illness.

Women and Men: What Are the Differences?

Biologically, women differ from men in several ways that are relevant to this discussion. Women are subject to unique organ-specific diseases and conditions (e.g., pelvic inflammatory disease [PID], endometriosis, uterine tumors, cervical cancer, and vaginal candidiasis), a higher incidence of some diseases (e.g., simple urinary tract infection, breast cancer, human papillomavirus infection [HPV]), and an increased likelihood of suffering serious consequences arising from common problems (e.g., gonorrhea, chlamydia).

Women die of complications related to pregnancy and to diseases of reproductive organs (e.g., cervical, breast, ovarian, and uterine cancers). The incidence of ectopic pregnancy (a pregnancy that grows outside of the uterus, usually in the fallopian tube) has increased dramatically since 1970. In 1970, one in 200 pregnancies was ectopic; in 1985, one in 48 was ectopic. This reflects, generally, an increase in sexually transmitted diseases (STDs). STDs such as gonorrhea and chlamydia often cause asymptomatic infection in women who later develop a condition called pelvic inflammatory disease. This acute problem often leaves scar tissue in the genital tract and greatly increases the risk of ectopic pregnancy, which in turn can rupture, causing hemorrhage and death.

Some studies note that women IVDUs experience more medical problems than male IVDUs. This probably reflects the broad spectrum of medical, social, and economic differences between men and women. All of this is important in understanding HIV infection in women.

Women and Symptoms

Are women's symptoms of HIV infection the same as or different from men's? Since we have little information related specifically to HIV disease in women, we have to look at other differences that can give us a basis for forming tentative answers to this question. Looking at the arena of STDs, we know that there are gendered differences in presentation (how symptoms show up medically, or "present"). In gonorrhea and chlamydia there is often a long silent phase in women (sometimes from three to six months), whereas men frequently show symptoms much sooner, such as a drip or burning during urination. Some bacterial infections often ascend to other organs in women (uterus, tubes), but rarely ascend in men. With monilia (yeast, or candida), trichomonas, and bacterial vaginitis, women frequently experience discharge, odor, itching, and pain while men often carry these organisms without any symptoms or medical consequences.

On the other hand, some sexually transmitted infections seem to be equally distributed and cause similar symptoms in men and women. Genital herpes and syphilis seem to have equal incidence sexually. With other infections that also cause sores or lesions on the genitals, the same type of symptoms occur with different frequency. More women and gay men are treated for warts (called condyloma, arising from HPV infection), and more men are seen clinically for chancroid (another ulcer-forming sexually transmitted infection of which there is increased incidence).

Another important difference is related to the menstrual cycle and vulnerability to infection. Many women with recurrent genital herpes report outbreaks with their periods. Other problems associated with periods include premenstrual syndrome (PMS) and toxic shock syndrome (which can be fatal). Hormone fluctuations result in recognizable changes in weight, fatigue, sexual desire, and so on.

A second issue concerning symptoms is whether or not the same symptom is viewed similarly in men and women. Are women's symptoms taken as seriously? It's not likely. Often women don't view their own health symptoms as seriously as they do others' symptoms. Mothers who are obviously ill themselves frequently come to a clinic or emergency room only when their children become sick. Many clinicians would probably interpret the same symptom—such as a headache—differently depending on a number of variables, including gender.

A review of the most common symptoms listed on health forms

from various HIV assessment programs that serve mainly male clients include fatigue, fever, chills, night sweats, weight loss, loss of appetite, headache, blurred vision, insomnia, confusion, concentration problems, sore mouth, sore throat, trouble swallowing, cough, shortness of breath, nausea and vomiting, diarrhea, muscle or joint pains, swollen glands, and skin changes. All of these symptoms could point to problems other than HIV illness, and many of them could be interpreted to reflect depression or psychological factors such as stress or overwork, which are diagnoses more often attributed to women. An HIV-positive woman, for example, may be at less risk for weight loss, because women have more body fat. Certainly weight loss is often ignored in women or understood inappropriately as something always favorable. There is simply no information regarding which symptoms different groups of HIV-positive individuals are most likely to experience. To improve early diagnostic capability and greater treatment availability for women, such studies must be undertaken. It is known that an early diagnosis can help prolong life if relevant medical services are available.

On the other hand, objective clinical signs that can be discovered by medical examination are much more likely to raise suspicion of HIV disease. Some frequent signs include specific medical conditions that can result in skin changes; mouth sores; findings on routine blood tests; and neurological changes such as problems with balance, numbness, or subtle changes in mental abilities. Yet practitioners who don't already have the eyebrow of suspicion raised often overlook clinical signs in women, especially since AIDS has, from the beginning, been defined as a gay men's disease. An obstetrician/gynecologist (ob/gyn) might find and treat a vaginal yeast infection after listening to a woman complain of discharge and itching. It is very unlikely that this doctor will then look in the client's mouth for oral signs of HIV disease such as herpes, thrush (oral yeast infection), hairy leukoplakia (an unusual growth associated with HIV disease), aphthous ulcers (canker sores), gingivitis (gum infection), or other medical conditions.

Male and Female Differences in the Mechanism of HIV Exposure

There are some clear differences between men and women in terms of sexual transmission of a variety of diseases. Where most STDs are concerned, women are often at greater risk than are men from a single episode of vaginal intercourse. For example, the risk of women being infected with gonorrhea is approximately double that for men. As repeated unprotected sexual intercourse occurs, the risks of transmission may be about equal. Still, a woman who has few sexual encounters with many men is at greater risk than a man who has few sexual encounters with many women; hence the biology of the double standard.

Exposure to HIV during sex does not always cause infection, but it is sometimes assumed that women are at greater risk than are men of exposure by heterosexual intercourse. There is evidence that in Africa and in the Caribbean the ratio of male-to-female cases of AIDS is about one to one. In recent studies of adolescents in New York City, this pattern of equal representation of women is now emerging. We need to know what variables increase a woman's risk of being infected. A woman with a chronic yeast infection or who is menstruating is at greater risk of *transmitting* HIV if she is infected, but is she also at greater risk of *contracting* HIV if she is not? It is this aspect of transmission that has not been studied or even considered, yet it suggests urgency for teaching risk reduction to women, whether heterosexual or lesbian. It is likely that a woman with an STD, a genital ulcer disease (herpes, chancroid, syphilis, lymphogranuloma venereum), condyloma (warts), or cervical dysplasia (an abnormal pap smear result) is at increased risk of acquiring HIV if exposed.

Some HIV transmission risks are equal for men and women, such as receiving anal sex and sharing intravenous (IV) drug works. But there are some unique risks when HIV-infected semen is deposited into the vagina. It is important to know that, while HIV has an affinity for T-lymphocytes (T-cells), it also can reside in other types of cells (other kinds of white blood cells, some types of neurological cells, and several others). The cells in the cervix are unique in that they respond to hormonal changes throughout a woman's cycle and play a significant role in allowing or disallowing different intruders to have access to the higher organs. An inhospitable cervix would never allow sperm to penetrate or pregnancy to occur. It is due to the cyclic change in immune function that these events are allowed to occur. The uterus and tubes are considered sterile and not to be invaded by ordinary or pathological germs, although "healthy" germs abound in the vagina (as they do in the mouth). The cervix, then, is a responsive organ, which has some power to decide what gets in.

In one small study of cervical tissue from HIV-positive women, the virus was able to be cultured from endothelial cells (lining of the cervix) and monocyte-macrophage cells (a type of white blood cell) as well as from the cervical mucus.[5] So, certain cervical cells actually become infected with HIV. In this study, the women with infected cells also had symptoms of an infected cervix (cervicitis). It is possible that HIV can cause a local cervicitis before spreading to the rest of the body. It is also likely that an already infected cervix is at greatly increased risk of becoming infected with HIV.

Further, in studies of the wart virus HPV, it has been found that, while the transmission rate is high for the virus (about 50 percent of sexually active heterosexuals test positive for HPV), the route by which viral expression and disease occur is not known. In fact, while nearly half of some samples are HPV positive, only 1.5 percent of women show clinical evidence of the warts.

Immune suppression in a woman's genital tract is proposed by some researchers as the mechanism of this phenomenon, and recurrent genital fungal and viral infections are associated with transient suppression of cell-mediated immunity.[6] Another proposed mechanism is an allergic response (to sperm, to yeast, to spermicides) inside the vagina, which may increase the likelihood of developing the warts. Allergic responses also relate to cellular immunity.

A good bit is known about immunity and women's genital tracts. It appears that cancer of the cervix, which is curable when detected early, often occurs following an invasion of microorganisms, particularly viruses. Whole books have been written on HPV and volumes regarding the minute details of cervical cancer, which is detected by routine pap smear screening. As yet, we have no proposed protocols for the gynecological care of HIV-positive women. Some of the research has been done; it simply hasn't been applied to understanding HIV infection.

About Opportunistic Infections

We know that HIV causes some life-threatening events as a viral agent. It is believed to be responsible for certain neurological (nervous system) disorders such as aseptic meningitis and AIDS dementia. But the majority of HIV-related problems occur because HIV suppresses the body's immune system: the reduced number and reduced capacity of lymphocytes make a person less able to fight infection. Almost all people will get ill when infected with certain harmful germs such as syphilis. The person whose immune system is compromised is at even greater risk of disease, complications, and death from such germs. But germs that are ordinarily harmless also threaten the lives of people who have HIV disease. Hence the term opportunistic infection.

Opportunistic infections are also caused by harmful germs that would normally cause only limited infection. For example, many healthy people have herpes sores on the lips at times, but when such herpes is found spreading to the throat or lungs in a person with HIV, it is considered opportunistic and is indicative of a damaged immune system.

Opportunistic infections that have been observed in men and women include coccidiodomycosis, cryptococcosis, cryptosporidiosis, isosporiasis, mycobacterium avium, mycobacterium Kansasii, M. tuberculosis, cytomegalovirus, pneumocystis carinii, toxoplasmosis, and candidiasis. These are the medical names for the bacteria, virus, fungus, protozoa, and so on that infect a compromised immune system. Ninety percent of AIDS deaths are attributed to opportunistic infections, many of which could be treated. Some opportunistic cancers are also associated with HIV disease, such as Kaposi's sarcoma (KS, which usually begins as a skin disease) and lymphomas (which begin in lymph tissue).

The frequency of both cancer and certain infections does differ by gender, but it has not been studied in relation to HIV disease. Women are known to have a very low incidence of KS, but are prone to chronic, persistent vaginitis. Beyond this, little is known regarding sex differences. There are known geographic differences in certain opportunistic infection prevalences, and the pattern of opportunistic infections in HIV disease differs greatly from patterns seen in other immunocompromised states, such as in people with cancer or on steroids. Young children with HIV disease get different opportunistic infections because their immune systems are both immature and compromised.

But the woman question? Well, it just hasn't been adequately studied.

Current Knowledge of Women's Genital Health Must Be Applied to HIV Disease

Information that can be obtained from medical texts, self-help books, and current research can be applied to the issues surrounding HIV disease.

Transmission issues seem to be related to vaginal health and therefore, naturally, to the practice of safer sex. Infections that go untreated probably increase the risk of HIV transmission to women. Genital tract health is affected by cyclic hormonal changes as well as by the types and combination of germs present in the vagina. Further exploration would probably reveal a unique pattern of opportunistic infection in the genital tracts of HIV-infected women. Some HIV-infected women may get sick and die of more ordinary infections such as chlamydia or monilia.

Chronic vaginitis, especially recurrent monilia or yeast infection, was noted in 24 percent of HIV-positive women in one study. Of these women, 86 percent progressed to AIDS.[7] Some researchers now suggest that chronic yeast is associated with a frequent incidence of oral thrush and is a good predictor for development of opportunistic infections. Research on whether such women would benefit from treatment of their vaginitis has not been undertaken.

What about other vaginal conditions? There has been a tremendous increase in the incidence of all STDs since 1980 in the United States, particularly of penicillin-resistant gonorrhea, syphilis, chlamydia, and herpes. Many such conditions lead to abnormal pap smears. Treating the infection often results in the return to a healthy cervix. Untreated or untreatable infections (such as herpes) often result in progression to cervical cancer—a known state of immunodeficiency. Some studies suggest that genital herpes (HSV-2) may be a risk factor for subsequent HIV infection in exposed men. At least 20 percent of women with visible warts on the cervix are found to have coexisting, precancerous changes. HIV infection, too, may be a risk factor itself for cervical changes that precede cancer. Women with HPV or genital herpes are told to have pap smears every six months. But we do not yet have guidelines on pap smear frequency for HIV-positive women.

Some Speculation about HIV Infection and a Woman's Body

Recognizing gender differences and understanding that HIV-positive women are dying without AIDS diagnoses suggest certain assumptions about what is going on in women who are exposed to HIV.

First, the mechanism of exposure differs where vaginal intercourse occurs. The cervix, which at certain times of the month allows sperm to travel into the uterus, is susceptible then in a unique way, at that time probably only surpassed by direct blood-to-blood transmission. So the rate of transmission may be high in a woman having unprotected vaginal sex with an HIV-positive man. Even in woman-to-woman sex, which many consider to be less risky, transmission risk is likely to be increased according to vaginal conditions. Any condition affecting the health of the vagina, genital tract, and rectum undoubtedly affects transmission rates and degree of exposure in all women.

Further, coexisting untreated infections render the vagina and cervix susceptible in additional ways.

When immunocompromise first occurs, an increase in STDs is likely. There is currently a dramatic increase in the rate of STDs, especially in teenage females who have had vaginal intercourse. Chronic, recurrent, difficult-to-treat infections are likely the next stage of early HIV infection. Young women without primary health care providers who are seen in emergency rooms probably get multiple doses of antibiotics, are not fully examined physically, and are probably not listened to regarding their complaints or believed when they say they took their medicine, did not have vaginal sex again, or whatever. Stereotypes abound among even the best health providers treating young women, including the assumption that all their patients are heterosexual, sexually active, unable or unwilling to follow directions, and so on.

In women who have tested positive for HIV antibodies, often a reversal of the above scenario occurs. The woman may complain of vaginitis on many occasions and be treated with vaginal suppositories without being given a pelvic exam. The provider may even know that candidiasis can occur vaginally in the HIV-positive female but know little else about the female genital tract. He or she may not be skilled at doing pelvic exams and may conduct an inadequate exam. Referrals are rare or nonexistent. Appropriate lab tests are often unavailable. This situation leaves an HIV-positive woman exposed to the continuing risk of the presence of multiple, known, and sometimes treatable infections and the additional risk of cervical cancer.

On the other hand, a known HIV-positive woman may seek and receive gynecological care and be treated adequately for gynecological problems by a provider who knows little about other subtle signs such as cough, weight loss, or oral thrush that may suggest early opportunistic infections. A woman with chronic lymphadenopathy and other signs may be diagnosed with ARC and end up dying of a pelvic infection that failed to respond to treatment. The failure to respond may indicate that the organism responsible for the infection was never identified. Some opportunistic infections that may in fact invade the upper genital tract include cytomegalovirus, tuberculosis, disseminated herpes, candida, and perhaps some of the rarer fungal infections. Certain other infections such as HPV might spread throughout the body or at least invade the upper genital tract under conditions of immunocompromise.

The shorter urethra in a woman exposes her urinary tract to more organisms from all kinds of sexual activity and even from certain hygiene practices (the anus, vagina, and urethra are all very close). Urinary tract infection by common germs and by opportunistic infections may occur more frequently in females than in males and must be studied. Chlamydia and gonorrhea in the pelvic organs may be more serious in HIV-positive women and may require different treatment, and opportunistic infections such as cytomegalovirus, M. tuberculosis, and salmonella may be involved.

Looking retrospectively at the deaths of women who were IV drug users or who died of pelvic infections or ectopic pregnancies, even reviewing maternal deaths to look for possible HIV-related signs, would probably be very revealing. One similar study in New York City on the deaths of male IVDUs revealed that a possible AIDS diagnosis had been overlooked in about half of the death certificates reviewed.

A Few Words about Research

Obviously much needs to be done. Educational materials need to be distributed to women and to doctors as well as to activists and social service workers. Research demands must be framed by activists, and research demands for women need to be framed by feminists. Women are suffering the medical effects of living in a sexist society.

We are important, we do get AIDS, we are not the same as men, we need our own place on the research agenda. And equally important, we must not be afraid to ask questions, undertake our own research projects, write about our experiences and about what we know. What we have to contribute to understanding the problem and having an impact on its solutions should not be underestimated.

Notes

1. Patricia Kloser, "Women with AIDS: A Continuing Study 1988," Newark, NJ: University of Medicine and Dentistry of New Jersey, in *V International Conference on AIDS: The Scientific and Social Challenge* (Ottawa, Canada: International Development Research Centre, 1989), p. 171.
2. John Piette, "Regional Differences in Survival with AIDS among Gay White Males in the United States," Providence, RI: Brown University, in *V International Conference on AIDS,* p. 170.
    Survival statistics vary greatly and can be difficult to interpret. It is clear, however, that race, gender, ethnicity, geography, incarceration, and drug use are all important variables that can affect survival time from diagnosis of AIDS to death from AIDS-related causes. Confounding these variables are the additional elements of access to care, appropriateness of care, adequacy of diagnostic ability, and accuracy of reporting.
3. Centers for Disease Control, *HIV/AIDS Surveillance Report,* January 1990, pp. 1-16.
4. Chris Norwood, "Alarming Rise in Deaths: Are Women Showing New AIDS Symptoms?" *Ms.,* July 1988, pp. 65-67.
5. R. J. Pomerantz et al., "Human Immunodeficiency Virus (HIV) Infection of the Uterine Cervix," *Annals of Internal Medicine,* 1988, Vol. 108, pp. 321-327.

6. F. H. Sillman and A. Sedlis, "Anogenital Papillomavirus Infection and Neoplasia in Immunodeficient Women," *Obstetrics and Gynecology Clinics of North America,* Vol. 14, no. 2, June 1987.
7. J. L. Rhoads et al., "Chronic Vaginal Candidiasis in Women with Human Immunodeficiency Virus Infection," *Journal of the American Medical Association,* Vol. 257, no. 22, June 12, 1987, pp. 3105-3107.

Additional references:

* T. W. Cheung and F. Siegal, "Kaposi's sarcoma (KS) in Women with Acquired Immune Deficiency Syndrome (AIDS)," Queens Hospital Center, Jamaica, NY, and Long Island Jewish Medical Center, New Hyde Park, NY. Presented at the V International Conference on AIDS, Montreal, June 1989.
* D. J. Gloeb, M. J. O'Sullivan, J. Efantis, "Human Immunodeficiency Virus Infection in Women," *American Journal of Obstetrics and Gynecology,* Vol. 159, no. 3, pp. 756-768.
* M. E. Guinan and A. Hardy, "Epidemiology of AIDS in Women in the United States 1981-86," *Journal of the American Medical Association,* Vol. 257, April 17, 1989, pp. 2,039-2,042.
* V. F. Holmes and F. Fernandez, "HIV in Women: Current Impact and Future Implications," *Physician Assistant,* May 1989, pp. 53-57.
* K. F. Kelley and S. H. Vermund, "Human Papillomavirus in Women: Methodologic Issues and Role of Immunosuppression," in *Reproductive and Perinatal Epidemiology,* M. Kiley, ed., Boca Raton, FL: CRC Press (forthcoming), 1990.
* C. Marte et al., "Need for Gynecologic Protocols in AIDS Primary Care Clinics," Bellevue Hospital, Community Health Project, New York, NY. Presented at the Fifth International Conference on AIDS, Montreal, June 1989.
* K. F. H. Miller et al., "High Rates of Cervical Dysplasias, Cervical Intraepithelial Neoplasias (CIN) and Human Papilloma Virus in HIV Infected Female Patients," Univeristy of Munich Women's Hospital, Munich, West Germany. Presented at the V International Conference on AIDS, Montreal, June 1989.
* H. Minkoff, "Confronting AIDS: What Every Woman's Physician Should Know," *Female Patient,* Vol. 12, 1987, pp. 49-64.
* J. L. Mitchell, "Women, AIDS and Public Policy," *AIDS and Public Policy Journal,* Vol. 3, no. 2, 1988.
* D. Ribble et al., "Difference in Stage of Presentation and Presenting Symptoms between Women and Men in a Primary AIDS Clinic," Bellevue Hospital, Community Health Project, New York, NY. Presented at the V International Conference on AIDS, Montreal, June 1989.
* R. W. Rochat et al., "Maternal Mortality in the United States: Report from the Maternal Mortality Collaborative," *Obstetrics and Gynecology,* Vol. 72, July 1988, pp. 91-97.
* R. Selik et al., "Impact of the 1987 Revision of the AIDS Case Definition in the United States," Centers for Disease Control, Atlanta. Presented at the V International Conference on AIDS, Montreal, June 1989.
* M. W. Vogt, D. J. Witt, D. E. Craven, "Isolation Patterns of the Human Immunodeficiency Virus from Cervical Secretions during the Menstrual

Cycle of Women at Risk for the Acquired Immunodeficiency Syndrome," *Annals of Internal Medicine,* Vol. 106, 1987, pp. 380-382.
- C. B. Wofsey, "Human Immunodeficiency Virus Infection in Women," *Journal of the American Medical Association,* Vol. 257, April 17, 1987, pp. 2,074-2,076.
- C. B. Wofsey et al., "Isolation of AIDS-Associated Retrovirus from Genital Secretions of Women with Antibodies to the Virus," *Lancet,* Vol. 1, 1986, pp. 527-529.

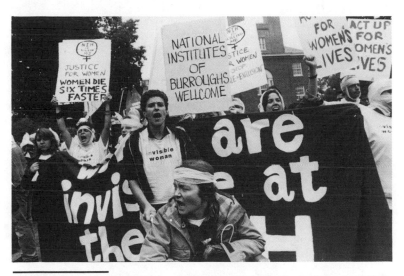

ACT UP protests at the National Institutes of Health in Bethesda, Maryland, May 21, 1990. The "Invisible Women," an affinity group, wore gauze to symbolize women's invisibility in AIDS research and treatment.

Photo by Donna Binder

Fighting for My Life

MELINDA SINGLETON

I am 35-years-old and I was diagnosed with HIV back in August of 1988, as having ARC, AIDS-related complex. I was an active drug abuser for two years, from 1980 to 1982, using heroin and cocaine with a needle. I got involved with IV drugs through my ex-boyfriend, who was an active user for many years. I also have a son, who is now 16-years-old. I just looked at myself in the mirror one day, and I decided it was time for me to go into a program and get some help. So I volunteered into a place called Good Samaritan. I did my treatment at the Highbridge Facility in the Bronx. I was the oldest female in treatment. I entered Good Samaritan in May of 1982 and graduated in May of 1984. During this time, my son was in South Carolina with his grandmother. I had brief conversations with him over the phone, but that was the extent of it. It was a very difficult situation, and feeling guilty about that was something that I worked very hard on in Samaritan.

I started to work in November of 1983 as a bookkeeper, and my boss promoted me. Six months later, I was managing a nice real estate firm in Manhattan. As soon as my son got out of school, I flew down to South Carolina and brought him back home to be with me again. It was a difficult reunion, a lot of anxiety, pain, and guilt. But it was good to have Samaritan, and groups, to try to work that out. I guess he needed reassurance, and he finally realized that Mommy wasn't going to mess up again, and that he was here to stay. He visited Samaritan, and was very, very proud of it, that Mommy did something to change her life.

I'm still very humble, and I'm still not very aggressive about some of the things that I deserve in life, but I have gotten a lot better. I've been going to therapy on my own to work on some of my insecurities as a woman and my feeling that I don't deserve a lot of things that I do deserve. With the help of my therapist, I was working on getting better things for me with my job—getting health insurance and more pay. I was somewhat afraid about asking for it. I thought, "At least I am working and I'm not using drugs, so, what the hell, that should be enough." But it wasn't. I deserve better.

So, with my therapist, I approached my boss back in May of 1988. I said, "Look, I need insurance for me and my son." Plus I was having some medical problems, and it was getting too expensive for me to pay out of my pocket. Then I said that I wanted a raise, and he said, "No problem. You just tell me what you want, and I'll get it for you."

So I contacted some insurance companies, and an agent came to my office. She asked me some basic questions, and filled out a form. Of course, the question of the drug abuse came up, and I denied it. She informed me that in a week or so some doctor would contact me to take my blood. This doctor called a couple weeks later. He came and took some of my blood, which I hate. I cannot stand needles to this day, after what they have done to me.

A couple of weeks later, I called my insurance broker and said, "Well, what happened with my insurance? Why is it taking so long?" She said, "Oh, I don't know. Let me check into it, and I'll get back to you." So she got back to me. She said that my insurance had been denied due to irregularities in my blood. So I said to my agent, "Well, what does that mean?" She said, "I'm sorry. The only person that can receive the information is your doctor."

I had to go above her head and call the main office. They told me that if I sent a fax to a certain person at their office, they would release the information to my doctor. So I ran out to a fax machine and wrote a letter saying that I authorized them to give the information regarding the irregularities in my blood to Dr. Levy, who was my doctor in the Bronx.

Well, that was about 3:00 in the afternoon, and I went back to my office and waited for Levy to call me. Couldn't figure out what in the world it could be. And at about 3:30, Dr. Levy called me and said, "Well, Melinda, I've got some bad news for you. You've got the AIDS virus. It was positive for AIDS." I said, "What are you talking about? You must be crazy. There must be a mistake." And he said, "No, there's no mistake. They take these special tests. You have to come into the office right away and get put on AZT."

Well, I flipped out. I started screaming and crying and told him they might have made a mistake and that I didn't want to talk to him, and I slammed the phone down in his ear. I called Carl, one of my tenants. He's an AIDS patient. I told him what had happened. He tried to calm me down. He said, first of all, that my doctor was a lunatic for ever telling me this over the phone. And second of all, it takes more than one test to get started on AZT. I got the AIDS hotline number and I called them up. After I don't know how many hours, I calmed down.

Levy did arrange for me to start taking AZT every four hours, 24 hours a day, as well as other medications. I had to buy three alarm clocks. I couldn't believe what was going on with my life.

I had to quit my job. Levy felt that for me to start leading a healthy life, I had to stop working and start taking care of myself. So my next project was to call my boss. I had to tell him, "I've got a problem. I'm not too well. I've got to stop working." He said, "What do you mean? What are you talking about?" I finally told him the truth. He felt that I was going to be OK. If I needed some time off, he would give it to me, but my job was always there for me, no matter what. And he said, "Don't listen to all these crazy doctors."

So I made an appointment with the Beth Israel Infectious Disease Clinic. And they sent me to the neurologist and the rheumatologist and the gynecologist and the Hospital of Joint Diseases, and every last one of them had a different approach to what was going on with me. I had cat scans and mammograms and EKGs, and I was put on all kinds of anti-inflammatories. And, in the meantime, they pulled me off all the AZT. I had to apply through a social worker for welfare. Suddenly, I went from making $30,000 a year and having a good job to being totally caught up in the system, in the bureaucracy of trying to get money for my son and myself. It was an absolute disaster.

I lost my therapist because they won't take Medicaid. So I got hooked up with another therapist. Suddenly I'm sitting in front of a new therapist, and I'm talking about the fact that I've got the AIDS virus. My perspective had changed. All the guilt about my son came back again, every last bit of the guilt that I worked all that time to get rid of. And the letdowns and the disappointments were all back again. I was back to blaming myself again. Once again, messing up. It was just awful.

Finally, my son confronted me about AIDS because of what he learned in school. He told me that I seemed just like somebody that has AIDS. I was trying to deny it, but I realized that it was just a question of time. So I sat down and told him that I was HIV positive, and that I had some arthritis, and some GYN problems, but that I was going to be fine. I just had to slow down a little bit, rest up, and get my system working again.

Every time you go to an appointment, to the doctor or to the clinic, they look at you and say, "Oh, but you don't look HIV positive. How did you catch it?" What am I supposed to say to them, I'm a dope fiend? I am an ex-dope fiend. So I tell them the truth.

I haven't been a drug fiend since 1982, and it still caught up with me. The doctors ask, "How much methadone do you take a day?" I say, "I don't take methadone, I told you. I'm drug free." They say, "I understand that drug addicts take methadone." "Some do, but I don't. Drug free, do you understand that?" They can't even comprehend the fact that I am drug free, that I don't have to be dependent on anything. That's a struggle. I just have to prove myself to everybody.

I heard about the Gay Men's Health Crisis, and I went and became a client of theirs. They treated me wonderfully. They gave me emergency money. They gave me all kinds of people to call. They gave me some of their newsletters about groups, and I started calling the hotline. I got the phone number of Women and AIDS Resource Network (WARN), where I got to speak to someone who was absolutely wonderful. I got information about something called Project Inform from California. And I started reading all these articles about HIV and different approaches to treatment. I also became involved, through the Hospital of Joint Diseases, with a group called People with Arthritis, who were also diagnosed HIV positive.

I was the only female everywhere I went. I went to a couple of Body Positive meetings; I was the only female. But I would go. I was determined to try to get my life back together again.

And I somehow found myself getting some control of my life again. I was scared to death every day, even of sneezing. I was afraid of getting sick. It was pretty rough. But I was trying to somehow regain some control of my life again. People were in and out of my house— visiting nurses, case workers. They wanted to see every piece of document of my life, from bank statements to records of everything that's happened to me. I felt like I was being analyzed under a microscope by the agencies of New York. I became very angry. I had worked all my life, paid taxes for this fucking country, and they weren't giving me nothing but a run-around.

I have a folder that you should see—hundreds of documents from different agencies, with questions and this and that. Thank God for the Gay Men's Health Crisis 'cause they've helped me out. I hadn't heard of any groups of women involved with AIDS.

I started strongly believing that I wasn't getting the proper treatment at all the different clinics I was going to. I was still taking a lot of medication. And I was trying to confront the doctors with some of the material that I had read. I got on the outs with some of the doctors. Complained about the GYN treatment. GYN was blaming IDC (Infectious Disease Clinic), IDC was blaming rheumatology, and nobody wanted to make any kind of decision. I said to myself, "Who is my primary physician?" Nobody seemed to be overlooking or reviewing my case. I feel like I'm getting thrown all these different pills from all these different places, and I'm just getting worse. I feel there's more that could be done for me and they're all barking up the wrong tree.

In the meantime, I'm just waiting for my disability, and I'm struggling, just trying to make it from one day to the next, with my rent and all kinds of things. Then they finally hooked me up with the Special AIDS Project for people with AIDS and ARC, and they started giving me some extra money and food stamps. They sent me a housekeeper to help me to clean my house and things like that. I let them to do that for awhile, but I didn't particularly like someone to come into my house, cleaning it, and digging around. I felt like I was imposed on enough about my privacy, something I value very highly. I loved my home, and I was very proud of it. I didn't like all these people in and out of there.

Things still weren't right, but I kept on seeing my therapist. I kept on working on it. And I kept on reassuring my son that his mommy was going to be fine. He seemed to be a bit more relaxed around me. He seemed to think that everything was going to be all right. He was showing me some of the pamphlets he got at school. Of course, you see it on TV all the time. You never hear anything positive. You always hear about all these damned people dying, and always, the deadly virus, and there's nothing mentioned about all the people who are out here surviving it, or finding better ways of making lives for themselves.

I kept on complaining to the doctors. I felt that, as a woman, they really didn't know what was going on with me. I'm full of cysts, I'm bleeding, and all these things. I guess they didn't know the answers. I was very unhappy with all of them.

I had to call the Hospital of Joint Diseases to tell them that the arthritis medication that they had me on wasn't doing a darned bit of good. I was in all this pain. I couldn't get up and down the stairs. I couldn't even carry my groceries anymore. It was ridiculous. They switched my medication, and tried this new one called Clinorel.

In the meantime, one of my tenants, who is also HIV positive, told me about his doctor, Dr. Schueller, and said that he was wonderful. Although he is in private practice, he does take Medicaid. I called

Dr. Schueller, and I went to see him. He looked at me with my cane, limping and carrying on, and he asked me about my history. I told him everything that had happened, and he shook his head and said, "You haven't had any physical therapy?" And I said, "Nope! Nothing. I've asked for it." And he said, "Well, give me some time, and I will try to work with you. And I'm sure that we can make things a lot better than what they are now." I signed consent forms with this doctor to get all my records transferred from all the other hospitals. In the meantime, I started feeling all achy and sore, and I was in so much pain. So I called him and he said to come back for an emergency appointment.

He took an X-ray, told me he thought that I was coming down with pneumonia, so he put me on a double dose of Bactrim. My son had just left for camp, for the summer. I started taking the Bactrim but I wasn't feeling any better. I couldn't even get up to get to work. So I went back to the hospital. They took some more X-rays, and said, "Oh, yeah, you've got pneumonia, PCP, and you're going to be here for awhile." I was scared to death. I said, "Oh, shit, here it comes." I lay in the emergency room for a few hours, and then another doctor came along and said I didn't have pneumonia. Well, to make a long story short, they admitted me.

I was so sick in the hospital. I started breaking out all over. And I was a disaster. I complained and complained. They had me on Bactrim. And they had me on IV. And they had me on painkillers and Tylenol with codeine. I was a wreck. I just couldn't hardly take it anymore. I was screaming at the doctors and in pain. Nobody understood what was going on with me. Within a couple of days, I looked like a monster. I had blisters all over my body, and I was quite sick. I had about 30 interns walking around, looking at me, poking at me. Then this old doctor said, "You don't know what's going on with her? She's having a severe allergic reaction to the medication you have her on. Take her off everything immediately, put her on lower dosages, and clean her out."

I didn't even have pneumonia at all. I was in the hospital for nothing to do with the HIV. Looking back, they did just exactly what I thought they were going to do. They overmedicated me instead of taking time to review what was going on. I mean, these motherfuckers nearly killed me from not paying attention to what was going on with me. And Schueller came in and said, "I'm so sorry. I messed up. I made a mistake. I forgot that you were taking Clinoril. And I'm afraid that the combination of Clinoril and Bactrim was what caused all of this."

I got up every day and made my own bed, tried to walk around. I lost, what, 15 pounds? But I fought with the doctors, and fought with myself to get up. A lot of my friends came by to see me. They brought me flowers. A lot of them looked at me as if I was fucking half dead already. I had lesions on my nose, and in my throat, and all over. I used to stand with cotton in the morning and try to unclog my eyes so I could see, because of the pus coming out of them.

I ended up in the hospital for three weeks. It was an experience that I don't ever want to wish on anybody. I was in a room with a big "blood precautions" sign on the door. It was awful. I felt like the nurses and the doctors wrote me off as another person with the AIDS virus, and that they weren't going to put too much time and effort into me, because I was going to be dying anyhow.

Anytime I start talking about the hospital, I get very angry. It took them four days before they even came in and started cleaning up my fucking room for me. I made my bed every day, but when I asked them to help wash me, they gave me a washrag in a bowl and said, "Do it yourself." I mean, they were disgusting. There is no excuse for the way they treated me, none whatsoever.

There was one nurse on duty who I'll never forget. She came in and took a look at the room, and said to the other nurses, "Clean this! And change this!" And she got me a special bed that was made out of air, because I had 80 or 90 percent lesions all over my body. She made it more comfortable for me, and she got me juices, and, oh, she was a sweetheart. Combed my hair for me, and made me feel a lot better. Of course, then she would go home, and that would be the end of it for the day, but at least there was something.

One of the interns took interest in me and realized that I had all intention of getting well, that I had not given up on life. He took me to the eye doctor because I almost lost my eyesight. That eye doctor wanted me to start taking medication right away. Well, nine hours after I saw him, I still hadn't gotten the medication. And I was in so much pain, my eyes were burning me, and my eyelashes had fallen off, and my eyebrows had fallen off. Then I called the patients' rights number, and they finally brought me my medication. It was like a battle every day to get them to treat me, and to show them that I was really going to beat this.

This was the first time I had ever been around any other women who had HIV like me. I was amazed at how uninformed they were about their situation—they knew nothing about diets or vitamins, or things they could do to better their lifestyles for themselves. They had social workers because they were on welfare. They all had been in the hospital for PCP at least once. They were surprised to hear about what I was telling them about different agencies that could help them with their children. All of them had children. It was very difficult for them to be home, being so sick all the time, with nobody helping them. I was very surprised. I told them to get in touch with their social worker while they were in the hospital, and get their social workers to help them. As a matter of fact, one of the women who came in didn't even have Medicaid. But they took her in anyhow. I guess that the system likes the fact that the less educated you are about your rights and your benefits, the more they can get over on you. I mean, it's a damned disgrace what they do to us. Women have been discriminated against all our lives. As long as I can remember, I've had to fight a battle for everything. They don't want to give you a job because you have kids, because they figure a woman will stay home and take care of the kids. I had to lie to get a job. The fact that I was living with my mother used to satisfy their fears that I wouldn't come to work.

The HIV situation is another story in itself. They say not to blame yourself, it's just some freak thing that's happened. But this freak thing that's happened has just totally disrupted my life. If I was in a relationship with a man right now, I don't think that I could make love and enjoy it, out of fear that somehow I could infect this person. We'd just have to find different ways of loving without having to make love. In my conscience and in my heart, I could not even enjoy it. Because I feel like there's a responsibility that goes with what I have. One of my biggest nightmares is that I'm going to be walking down the street, or riding the subway, and some dummy is going to stab me. All these people are running up to help me. And I have to tell them, "No, no, no, you can't help me! I'm HIV positive! No, don't touch me! I don't want you to touch my blood!" And I lie there and I bleed to death because I have this tremendous responsibility on my shoulders to make sure I don't get anybody exposed to the HIV.

There should be more research done for women. I mean, I have multiple cysts on my ovaries. I've got irregular bleeding all the time. I've got multiple cysts on my breasts. But I'm not taking any kind of medication right now, ever since that happened with that allergy reaction. I'm scared to death of taking anything. I am taking this inhalator because I'm having severe breathing problems, and they say I have asthma or allergies or bronchitis. Well, I think they're full of shit. I think my lungs got damaged when I was in the hospital, from all the lesions on my lungs, and the pentamadine they were giving me intravenous before they realized that I didn't have PCP. Who knows?

When I walked out of the hospital, I was down to 116 pounds. I got up to 130 pounds again, on my own. I read nutritional books, special diets, took multiple doses of vitamins. I listen to these tapes now to try to learn to meditate and stop smoking. I'm still seeing Dr. Schueller. Everybody tells me I should be suing him. But if I sue him, I should sue the whole world for everything they've put me through. Schueller's just part of this thing.

He's amazed at how I have bounced back, at how beautiful my skin is. Well, it's no thanks to any of them; it was me. I'm working now, off the books. I feel good getting up and dressed every day, doing some work and feeling somewhat constructive with my life. I'm getting disability, and I don't feel a bit guilty about taking it. I've paid Social Security and taxes for 25 years. I have a 16-year-old son whom I have to send to school, and have things for, and clothe and feed.

The reason I'm saying all this is because it took me a whole damned year to understand everything that's happened. The medical profession needs to do some research about women with AIDS. My Social Security caseworker admitted to me that they're not quite sure how to treat women's AIDS claims that are coming in. We don't fall into the categories that the gay men do; our illnesses are somewhat different. No doctor will say, "This is because of HIV" or "This isn't because of HIV"; they don't know. I do think that my female problems are definitely related to this HIV, but, no, I don't have KS [Kaposi's sarcoma] and some of the other things that most people think of as the signs of AIDS. But that does not mean that I'm not having problems.

I still feel that with a healthy attitude, good moral support, and doctors who will take interest in you and try to work with you and discuss your case, you can stay relatively healthy. I mean, we're talking about my life. Who are they to play guessing games? I have the right to make decisions as to what medications I feel might be helpful, especially if I show an interest and am willing to work with them. They treat me like an imbecile or some poor soul. I've watched them at the hospital, and I've been so angry with them sometimes. The average attitude is, "Ah, let's just make them comfortable"; they just write you off, because you're gonna die anyhow, so what the hell? I don't agree with that attitude at all. I don't. And I'm going to be around for quite some time. It's a hell of a struggle to always have to prove yourself. If I had cancer, they'd be all over me, trying to do all these things for me. But with the AIDS virus, it's a whole different approach from the beginning to the end.

We're no less human because of the HIV or because we're women. None of us deserve to have this. None of us. No matter what the circumstances were. It's not right. And we're going to have to change it.

HIV-Antibody Testing and Legal Issues for HIV-Positive People

ZOE LEONARD

What is commonly known as the "AIDS test" is a test for the presence of HIV antibodies in the blood. There is some controversy in the medical and AIDS communities as to whether HIV is the cause of AIDS or only a cofactor.[1] However, there has been enough statistical correlation between HIV and immune suppression to take test results seriously. People who test HIV positive are thrown into a medical, emotional, and legal limbo. They need a range of medical and social services to which they may not have access. It is through the test that many people first confront their fears of illness and death. And, though the test result itself does not indicate an AIDS diagnosis, it can lead to harassment, discrimination, and ostracism. Some testing issues affect women specifically, such as calls for mandatory testing of pregnant women.

Testing is not treatment or prevention, and cannot take the place of either. The test is an effective tool only if it is accompanied with education and access to treatment. There is a difference between testing and screening. Screening is a public health measure which applies the HIV-antibody test to populations with the intention of prevention of transmission or epidemiological surveillance. Testing is the use of the test on an individual basis. When an individual chooses to get tested, she or he is making a decision, usually based on a desire to seek treatment or to face fears of infection.

This section outlines a sane approach to testing regarding both personal decision making and public policy-making.

The Test

There is no such thing as an "AIDS test." What is currently available is an HIV-antibody test. In most situations, an enzyme-linked immunosorbent assay (ELISA) test is done first. If it is positive twice, a more sensitive confirmatory test is done, usually the Western Blot. Both these tests determine if you have been infected with HIV by indicating whether or not you have antibodies to the virus in your blood. When you are exposed to a virus, your body develops antibodies to that specific virus.[2] Since the test responds to the antibodies rather than the virus itself, it is advisable to wait at least a few weeks after your last possible exposure to HIV. Most people will develop measurable amounts of antibodies within a few weeks of exposure, but it can take up to 18 months.[3]

After you take the test, you will have to wait from a few days to a couple of weeks for your results. A lot of people are very nervous about getting their results, so you might want to bring a friend with you, and make sure that you have time afterwards to talk about it. Even if you are negative, the process can be emotionally draining.

Accuracy

There are a certain number of false positives, so if you test positive you may want to retest. There is no stable, predictable percentage of false positives, but they occur more frequently in older people, intravenous drug users (IVDUs), and women who are pregnant, have had many children, take certain medications, or have certain chronic illnesses. Inconclusive results occur in 1 to 8 percent of all tests.[4] If your Western Blot test results are repeatedly inconclusive, the lab can do an immunofluorescent assay, another confirmatory test.

False negatives are extremely rare as long as enough time has passed for the person to develop antibodies.

A Negative Result

A negative result means that the test has not detected any antibodies to HIV in your blood. This probably means that you have not been exposed to the virus, but you could have been infected and not yet developed the antibodies. After testing negative, if you consider yourself at risk or are displaying symptoms, the standard recommendation is that you wait six months, avoid all risky behavior, and retest. If both your first and second test results are negative, then you probably have not been exposed to HIV, but remember it can take up to 18 months to seroconvert (change from HIV negative to HIV positive). Testing negative does not mean you are immune! You are as vulnerable to infection as you were before you got your results, and can still be infected if you come into contact with HIV. It is still important to follow safe-sex and safe needle-use guidelines.

A Positive Result

A positive result indicates that you are infected with HIV. It does not mean that you have AIDS, it does not mean that you have to stop having sex, it is not a death sentence. It's not certain that all HIV-positive people will progress to AIDS. Many people remain HIV positive but asymptomatic and healthy for years.

Being infected with HIV means that you can infect other people regardless of whether you are currently well or sick. Safe sex and not sharing drug works are essential to protect your partners. You also need to protect yourself against reinfection. Multiple exposures increase the amount of virus that your body will then have to fight.

It is important that you assess your overall health, especially the health of your immune system. It helps to find a physician or a clinic that is knowledgeable about HIV infection. Have a complete physical and a blood work-up, including marker tests that indicate the level of viral activity. Talk to your doctor about your treatment options. There is no cure for AIDS, but you can fight it more effectively if you know the condition of your body.

Testing positive can be overwhelming and depressing. Many people have found it to be very traumatic, and some have even attempted suicide. While the difficulty of receiving a positive test result should not be underestimated, it is helpful to recognize that many people have been able to make positive changes in their lives, such as stopping drug use and creating supportive relationships. Try to get as much support and help as possible—medical, emotional, financial, and legal. You might want to find a support group or counseling. The goal is to find a middle road, understanding and acting on the dangers of HIV infection without panicking.

Besides having medical and emotional consequences, a positive test may also result in harassment and discrimination, some of it legal, some illegal. Discrimination issues are discussed later in this section.

Making Your Decision

The illnesses associated with HIV infection are so serious, and HIV-infected individuals are so stigmatized by factions of our society, that there is a tremendous amount of anxiety around being tested. The decision to take the test is a difficult one.

A few years ago, when there were no promising drugs available, many people felt there was no point in testing unless you were sick enough for hospital care. Now there are medical reasons to test: drugs such as AZT and pentamidine may effectively fight off opportunistic infections. Improving your diet, work habits, and mental attitude, and coping with stress are also important aspects of fighting HIV disease. The sooner you can begin to deal with an HIV-positive status, the better your chances are for long-term survival.

Testing needs to be part of a system that includes health care and social services. Government and certain private institutions push testing rather than put money into treatments, drug trials, and education. It is necessary to fight for better medical care and more access to the existing network of organizations and individuals who can help.

Some people feel they need to know their status for very personal reasons. Psychologically or spiritually, they just need to know. You may want the relief of knowing after a long period of doubt, or you may want to reorganize your life with your HIV status as a consideration.

Another reason to test is that you might be HIV negative, which can be an enormous relief. If you took the test because you were sick, you can now rule out HIV as a cause and get a more accurate diagnosis.

Some people choose not to test. They may not want to deal with the stress of knowing. One responsible way to approach this is to assume that you are positive and to behave accordingly by always practicing safe sex, and taking care of your overall health.

The Importance of Anonymity, Counseling, and Informed Consent

If you decide to take the test, it is important to make sure the test is administered in the best possible situation. It is crucial that you have pre- and post-test counseling. This counseling allows you to ask questions of a knowledgeable person when you get your results. Testing should never be done without education and counseling. Often, private physicians are not equipped to provide proper counseling, or they may not take the time. Physicians and researchers doing seroprevalence studies may offer free testing or even pay for blood samples from people they consider to be at "high risk," but they rarely offer any kind of counseling at all. It's not worth it. Make sure you get counseling with your test.

Anonymous testing is the safest way to find out HIV status. There are centers that provide free, anonymous HIV-antibody testing with pre- and post-test counseling. In an anonymous test, you never give your name; you are identified only by a number. This way, the decision of whether, to whom, how, and when to reveal your test result is left up to you. It is your own responsibility to tell anyone you may have infected, and to protect future partners from infection. We need more anonymous testing centers—currently the waiting list can be weeks long.

A positive test result could affect your job, housing, and relationships with other people. "Confidential" testing is available, but it is different from anonymous testing. In a confidential test, your name is used and the results are put into your medical records. A positive HIV test could result in denial of insurance coverage. In most of the United States, anonymous testing is available. In states where it is not, some people have crossed into other states in order to test anonymously.

Most states require "informed consent" to ensure that proper pretest counseling has taken place. You may be asked to sign a form, stating that you are not being coerced to take the test. Although this is good in theory, you should never be required to give your name. If you are signing something with your name, then you are getting a confidential test, not an anonymous one.

Home testing kits may be available soon. They are not a good idea because there is no counseling, and the rate of false positives is not yet known. Florida already prevents their sale.

Mandatory Testing and Screening

There are circumstances under which you are not allowed to make any decisions about testing. If you are in the military, applying for citizenship, or a member of certain "special populations," you may find yourself being tested against your will, having your status reported to the department of health, or, in a worst case scenario, being quarantined.

Much of the government's focus on the AIDS crisis has been to identify, isolate, and punish HIV-infected people rather than offering them treatment, housing, and support. Massive screening has taken place without any logical use for the data collected. Screening programs are justifiable by public health standards only when an affordable, effective, safe treatment is available to those who are positive. If the same money and time were used for education, free anonymous test sites, counseling, and early interventions for HIV-positive, asymptomatic individuals, we would all be healthier and better informed.

Federal Screening Programs

The federal government has an enormous screening program. The Defense Department screens all new recruits and active duty personnel. New recruits and ROTC students who test HIV positive are not permitted to enter the military. There is no requirement that HIV-positive personnel be discharged, but there are severe penalties for homosexuality and drug use, and people are often harassed or discharged on those grounds. Perhaps this is why such a high percentage of men in the military have claimed to have been infected by prostitutes.

In addition, the State Department and Peace Corps screen foreign service personnel. The State and Defense Departments' policies have been upheld by the courts, but the screening program used by the Job Corps, a training program for underprivileged inner-city kids, is being challenged by Lambda Legal Defense Fund.[4]

Anyone applying to immigrate to the United States is screened, and HIV-positive individuals are not allowed permanent residency or citizenship. Those who already have residency and are applying for citizenship need not test, and those applying under the amnesty program can often get waivers. However, the waiver option is not well publicized, so those who think they may be HIV positive remain undocumented and ineligible for health care that is afforded to citizens. Fear of discrimination and deportation drives many people underground.

All federal prisons screen inmates.

State Screening Programs

Many states have enacted legislation that mandates compulsory screening in many "special populations," including applicants for marriage licenses, pregnant women, newborns, hospital patients, mentally ill or mentally retarded patients, prisoners, prostitutes, IVDUs, and sex offenders. Some states reserve the right to test any individual "suspected" of being an "AIDS carrier," and so allow for harassment. New legislation is being passed constantly. The major problem with these programs is the focus on testing rather than on prevention, education, treatment, and protection of civil rights.

Premarital screening: Legislation requiring that all who apply for marriage licenses be tested for HIV antibodies has been proposed in almost every state. Several states require that all applicants get information and an option to test. Utah prohibits and declares void any marriage with a person who has AIDS. In 1987 Illinois enacted a law requiring an HIV test for anyone being issued a marriage license. Before the law was repealed in 1989, only 52 people, out of 250,000 applicants, were HIV positive. One study estimated the cost of this screening program at $60,000 to $100,000 per case found, and that 26 percent of these "cases" were false positives.[5]

Prenatal and postpartum testing: Florida and Michigan require pregnant women to test for HIV. New York and New Jersey are considering legislation that would require testing of all pregnant women, newborns, and postpartum mothers. The Centers for Disease Control (CDC) recommends that pregnant women in "high-risk groups" be tested.

Patients: In cases where health care or emergency workers think they may have been exposed to HIV by needlestick injuries or other contact with a patient's body fluids, some states will force the patient to be tested.

Texas and Wisconsin authorize compulsory screening of mentally ill or mentally retarded residents in state facilities. "Incompetent" persons may be tested without consent in Washington. Rhode Island, much more sensibly, requires health care professionals to offer an HIV test in hospitals and family planning, prenatal, and sexually transmitted disease (STD) clinics, but does not allow testing without informed consent.

Prisoners: Screening of inmate populations in state prisons has usually been initiated by prison administrators rather than legislators. However, as of November 1988, 14 state prison systems had mass screening programs; 28 states segregate prisoners with AIDS or ARC, or HIV-positive prisoners.[6] Although these prisons insist on testing, they do not provide treatment or dental dams and condoms for safer sex for inmates.

Persons charged with or convicted of certain offenses: Many states authorize testing if there is a charge or conviction of sexual assault, rape, prostitution, sale or use of illegal drugs, or any crime where there might have been needle sharing or sexual contact. California, Iowa, Rhode Island, and Washington authorize testing of persons charged with assault involving spitting, scratching, biting, or "lewdness." These laws do not require the individual to be convicted, but only charged with a crime. If we support anonymous voluntary testing, we must support it for all people, even those convicted of sex crimes.

Licensed prostitutes: In Nevada, the only state that regulates prostitution, all prostitutes must submit to HIV testing. It is a felony for a prostitute to work after she or he is informed of a positive test result. These laws do not distinguish between high-risk sex (unprotected intercourse) and no-risk sex (hand jobs). The owner of a house of prostitution is liable for any "third-party damages" resulting from a seropositive employee. One of the dangers of enforcing mandatory testing and quarantine of HIV-positive sex workers is that the johns might then assume that all infected women have been isolated, and will then be reluctant to use condoms. This leaves women sex workers vulnerable to HIV transmission from HIV-positive johns who either don't know or don't care about their own serostatus and won't use condoms.

Demands

- Free anonymous testing in every state.
- More test sites.
- Pre- and post-test counseling required with each test.
- Proper testing procedures for participants in research studies.
- No mandatory testing.

Legal Issues

The legal and ethical issues that arise when one analyzes HIV-antibody testing lead to a much broader discussion of AIDS-related law. The goal of public health law should be to safeguard the health of all citizens. Yet many AIDS laws are based on irrational fear, bigotry, and narrow definitions of morality, rather than on sound medical facts and effective models of prevention. Politicians often respond to political pressure rather than to public health concerns and have enacted dangerous and shortsighted legislation such as authorization of compulsory screening, quarantine, and criminalization of HIV transmission.

The 1988 "Helms Amendment" shows how the law can frustrate rather than facilitate effective educational efforts. The amendment forbids the funding of any AIDS prevention programs that "promote or encourage...homosexual or heterosexual activity..." This and other rulings that require that abstinence be stressed rather than safe sex are unrealistic when discussing a virus that can be sexually transmitted.

HIV Reporting

All states require reporting of AIDS cases (as defined by the CDC) to the public health department. A growing number of states require reporting of HIV-positive test results. Although confidentiality is required, there have already been problems. In South Carolina, test results have been revealed, and individuals have lost their jobs due to discrimination.[7]

Many states allow for anonymous testing sites but require names under certain circumstances. Oregon, for example, requires the names of seropositive infants and people who indicate they will not notify their partners.[8] If people have to give their names, they are less likely to test, and are therefore more likely to infect others and to go longer without obtaining treatment.

Isolation

Laws that provide for quarantine operate on the assumption that infected people must be separated from the "general population." In the case of HIV, which is not transmitted through casual contact, a desire to separate and punish certain people (homosexuals, drug users, and/or prostitutes) may be the underlying motivation for quarantine initiatives. Some states authorize isolation for all sexually transmitted or communicable diseases and include HIV infection in these categories. Other states have passed new, HIV-specific legislation.

No state at this time is quarantining all HIV-positive individuals, but some states now authorize quarantine of "recalcitrant" individuals. This can mean anyone who has sex after testing positive for HIV, even though the laws do not usually differentiate between no-risk and high-risk sex. The wording allows for a highly subjective definition of responsible behavior for any individual. These laws can be enforced selectively and used as tools to harass "social undesirables."

Isolation is punishment without a crime—it does not require criminal conviction, but is based on potential future actions. Because there is currently no cure for HIV infection, quarantine would basically amount to a life imprisonment sentence.

Isolation may prevent risky behavior in certain individuals, but as a health policy it would have negative impact. With the threat of quarantine, far fewer people are likely to test voluntarily or seek treatment for HIV disease. Punitive measures have not been successful in controlling sexually transmitted diseases in the past, and in fact are more likely to result in an increase rather than a decrease. Fear of discrimination drives people underground.

Crimes of Transmission

In many states it is now a crime to transmit HIV knowingly. The charges and penalties vary widely. Some laws allow criminal prosecution for spitting, biting, and scratching, which are unproven and unlikely to transmit HIV. Almost no laws require proof of transmission or seroconversion. Several cases involved convictions based on "intent to commit harm" by transmission through saliva, despite its medical implausibility. In 1989, Gregory Scroggins was charged with attempted murder and received a ten-year sentence for biting a cop, although the officer in question has repeatedly tested negative. In Texas, a man is serving a life sentence for spitting at a prison guard. In Kansas, a man spat on two officers and was charged with six felonies, including "making a terroristic attack." In Indiana, a PWA who was attempting to commit suicide was charged with attempted murder because he bit, spat at, and splashed bloody water at emergency medical workers.[9] Public health policy must be based on medical fact, rather than on unfounded fears about implausible means of transmission.

Some laws do pertain to proven methods of transmission. In Georgia, for example, people who know they are HIV positive and perform any sexual act without revealing their status face sentences of up to ten years regardless of whether or not latex barriers were used. The same law covers needle sharing, agreeing to have sex for money, or donating blood. It is highly problematic for the law to intervene in consensual sex or needle sharing. How can it be proven that the person knew their status, understood what it meant, and understood how HIV is transmitted? When sex is consensual, both parties bear responsibility. It is difficult to understand what went on in a private interaction. When sex is not consensual—in cases of rape or sexual abuse—the person being raped has no opportunity to protect herself or himself, or to negotiate safer sex; the rapist bears full responsibility. Currently, many states require HIV testing of all persons charged with (not necessarily convicted of) sex crimes. Not only is testing not always warranted, depending on the specific circumstances, but the civil liberties of all individuals deserve protection. Prevention cannot be punitive in nature. The only effective way for people to safeguard their health is by having the right information and the self-respect to use it.

Contact Tracing

Contact tracing is a form of medical surveillance that seeks the sexual partners of an "index case" (infected person) and informs them that they may have been exposed to a sexually transmitted disease. Contact tracing depends on the index case's knowing, remembering, and wanting to give the names of all his or her sexual contacts for up to ten years. Many states have contact tracing programs. Some see it as a "solution" to the AIDS crisis, but it is perhaps the most expensive and least effective way of stopping the spread of HIV. The money used for contact tracing comes out of limited resources allotted to AIDS and public health. We need free anonymous testing, counseling, education, and treatment, not a growing list of names.

Fighting Discrimination

Many people are afraid to find out their antibody status because of the discrimination they may face if they test positive for HIV antibodies. Discrimination can occur in all areas of our lives, including loss of employment, loss of housing, disqualification from insurance benefits, exclusion from school, disinheritance, denial of visitation rights in hospitals, and loss of child custody, among others. Because much of the government and mass media's information about HIV/AIDS focuses on "risk groups," discrimination is not limited to people with AIDS (PWAs) but can also be directed towards people who are perceived to be sick or in a "high-risk group."

Most protection against discrimination is now legislated on a state or local level; some states provide no protection at all. Federal law supersedes state and local laws, or lack thereof. Section 504 of the Federal Rehabilitation Act of 1973 provided some protection from discrimination against the disabled, including PWAs, but only by federally funded institutions.

The Americans with Disabilities Act, passed in 1990, extends the protections of Section 504 to the private sector, prohibiting discrimination based on perceived or actual disability, including HIV infection, in the areas of public accommodation, housing, and employment. It was long delayed in Congress because the language makes clear that HIV infection is to be included as a disability, and because the bill mandates that all doctors' and dentists' offices are to be considered public accommodations. This means that no HIV-positive person can be refused treatment because of his or her HIV status.[10]

Individual cases of discrimination have been successfully fought by civil rights and gay and lesbian groups, including Lambda Legal Defense Fund, the American Civil Liberties Union, and the AIDS Discrimination Unit of the New York City Human Rights Commission, among others.

Insurance

The insurance industry demonstrates clearly the inadequacy of a system which provides health care for profit. PWAs, HIV-positive people, and those considered to be at "high risk" are seen as bad gambles by insurance companies; therefore, it is increasingly difficult for large numbers of people to get health, disability, or life insurance.

Since health insurance is not closely regulated, insurance companies and employers who provide health coverage have been getting away with highly discriminatory practices. Insurance companies have regularly denied coverage to disabled people and people with chronic illnesses; they are now also denying coverage to people with HIV infection. Some companies require an HIV test and exclude applicants who test positive. Others reject applicants with a history of sexually transmitted disease, and many ask if you, or anyone in your family, has a history of IV drug use. Some companies have gone so far as to reject applicants on the basis of marital status, occupation, or even zip code.

Even people who already have medical coverage are not necessarily secure: insurance companies are now placing ceilings on the amount they will pay for AIDS care. Others are making wide use of "preexisting condition" clauses, making the most of HIV infection's long incubation period. It is also common practice to refuse payment for many AIDS treatments because they are still categorized as only experimental.

One company, Galaxy Carpet Mills, has written a clause into its employees' health policy which limits medical reimbursements for people with AIDS or other sexually transmitted diseases, unless they can prove they were "involuntarily acquired"; if the employee was infected through needle sharing or sex, he or she is not entitled to full medical benefits. In 1988, another company, Circle K, denied benefits to all new employees with AIDS—except those who contracted HIV through a blood transfusion, and women who "unknowingly" contracted HIV from their husbands.[11] Both companies' policies were finally rescinded after much public protest, coordinated nationwide by ACT UP and other activist groups. The idea of distinguishing between "voluntary" and "involuntary" infection is just a new wording of an old bigotry.

Demands

- No contact tracing.
- No quarantine or isolation of HIV-positive people or PWAs.
- Prohibition against discrimination by insurance companies, employers, landlords, schools, or health care providers against gay men, lesbians, HIV-positive people, PWAs, or people with other disabilities.

Notes

1. Some people have died of AIDS without ever testing positive for HIV antibodies.
2. Unlike other virus' antibodies, HIV antibodies do not provide adequate defense against the virus.
3. Paul Hardings and Laura Pinsky, *The Essential AIDS Fact Book* (New York: Simon & Schuster, 1989).

4. David Barr, Lambda Legal Defense Fund, personal communication, November 1989.
5. Larry O. Gostin, "Public Health Strategies for Confronting AIDS: Legislative and Regulatory Policy in the U.S.," *Journal of the American Medical Association*, Vol. 261, no. 11, March 17, 1989.
6. Gostin, "Public Health Strategies."
7. DiAna DiAna, South Carolina AIDS Education Network, personal communication, November 1989.
8. *State AIDS Reports* No. 7, State AIDS Policy Center, George Washington University, February-March 1989.
9. Robert Massa, "The Skin of our Teeth," *Village Voice,* December 26, 1989.
10. Steven A. Holmes, "The House Approves Bill Establishing Broad Rights for Disabled People," *The New York Times,* May 23, 1990, p. A1.
11. Marguerite Holloway, "The No-Fault Health Policy," *Village Voice,* January 9, 1990.

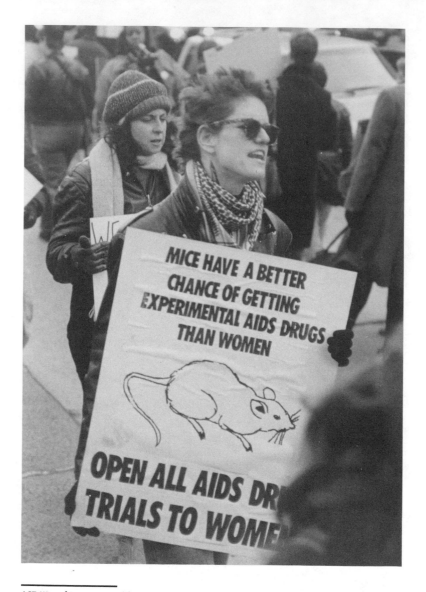

ACT UP and Women's Health Action and Mobilization (WHAM) demand the inclusion of women, people of color, and IVDUs in experimental drug trials at the New York University AIDS Clinical Trial Units, on International Women's Day, March 8, 1990.

Photo by Miriam Lefkowitz

Treatment and Trials

RISA DENENBERG

The current health care delivery system cannot meet the challenge posed by the AIDS crisis. In large urban areas where drug addiction, tuberculosis, homelessness, and HIV illness are common, there are not enough hospital beds. People wait days for treatment in emergency rooms, and a significant portion of the population does not seek treatment because it cannot pay for needed health care services. Health care delivery is stratified (rich to poor), fragmented (lacking in an overall plan), and specialized (different doctors for different body parts) rather than centering on the individual as a whole person. The AIDS crisis is foremost an economic problem. Health care for people with AIDS is based on a paradigm that suggests that only white, gay men get AIDS. Not even white, gay men are getting decent health care, and everyone else is lost within this epidemic. Primary health care, a holistic perspective, and socialized medicine are three useful concepts in considering the scope of changes needed in the current system.

Primary health care means a health care provider has an ongoing, caring relationship with a patient over time, making referrals to specialists as needed, while maintaining active involvement in health care planning. Holistic health care considers an individual in a total way, with a concern for emotional, physical, social, sexual, and spiritual health.

Socialized medicine, also called universal health care, while not necessarily a panacea, ensures that each individual in a society has access to the existing health care system and equal access to available services and treatments.

In the arena of HIV illness, adequacy of treatment should be measured by additional standards. These elements make up the optimal standard of treatment:

- Clinicians maintaining up-to-date knowledge of all available AIDS treatments and their adverse effects for all populations affected by AIDS. This includes knowing how AIDS drugs will affect a woman's reproductive system and interact with other drugs such as methadone. Adverse effects range from the treatment being highly toxic to being prohibitively priced.
- Agreement between the patient and clinician to monitor the patient's health at appropriate intervals for the duration of the condition, monitoring all indications of illness (called markers) including, and most important, quality-of-life issues.
- Prophylaxis (preventive treatment) for all likely opportunistic infections.
- Respect on the part of clinicians for the patient's participation in her own health care and willingness to provide care regardless of which therapies a patient chooses or refuses, including alternative therapies such as acupuncture, macrobiotics, or herbal remedies.

Markers of HIV Disease

Markers are laboratory tests that give information about the course of disease, in much the same way that taking the temperature gives some indication of how sick someone is. The primary marker in HIV disease is the T-cell (a type of lymphocyte or white blood cell) count. T4 (CD4 or helper)-cells and T8 (CD8 or suppressor)-cells are counted and compared as a ratio. A decrease in T4-cells and a decrease in the T4/T8 ratio are often associated with acceleration of HIV disease. Serial tests, although expensive, must be undertaken for the information to be meaningful. T-cell counts are frequently used as a basis for planning medical treatment; for example, initiating antiviral medications or prophylaxis against pneumocystis carinii pneumonia (PCP).

Other clinical markers in use include HIV p24 core antigen, beta-2 microglobin, and neopterin. P24 appears early, may disappear, and then occur later in the course of illness. Linked with a drop in T4-cells, the reappearance of p24 may predict a rapid progress to AIDS.

Beta-2 microglobin is a protein shed from HIV-infected cells, and increases may suggest disease progress. Neopterin, a product of macrophages (another type of white blood cell), can be measured in blood or urine as a nonspecific indicator of HIV infection. New tests are being developed. Of particular interest are tests of virus levels in serum (the fluid left in a blood sample after all of the cells are removed). It is hoped that this will prove to be a more sensitive, more direct marker for staging HIV illness and evaluating treatments.

It is important to understand that laboratory markers cannot fully describe a person's health status. Like all biological tests, their meanings are subject to interpretation. Also, it is important to recognize that the usefulness of laboratory markers has been observed primarily in white men. Therefore, their applicability to women and all people of color cannot be assumed to be valid. Further investigation is warranted. Other indicators of well-being such as weight maintenance, good energy levels, lack of symptoms, and the ability to function as usual may be more important measures of health and also must be monitored by health practitioners.

State-of-the-Art HIV/AIDS Treatment

Medical management of an HIV-positive, asymptomatic client enrolled in a community clinic or seeing a private doctor would likely include frequent visits for physical exams and laboratory work. Lab studies would serially follow markers of HIV illness such as T-cells, p24 antigen, and beta-2 microglobin. Vaccinations (e.g., hepatitis, flu shots, pneumococcal pneumonia) would be brought up to date and maintained. Periodic testing for tuberculosis would be conducted. Identification and treatment for any opportunistic infection would be initiated at early stages. Problematic symptoms would be treated with medication, diet, or other strategies. Emotional well-being would be supported. Nutritional advice and access to a social worker would be available at the same site. Current therapies would be explained and offered at the joint decision of provider and client. Approved antivirals (AZT and/or acyclovir) may be started. If so, frequent visits to monitor side effects, such as anemia, would occur. Prophylaxis to prevent PCP would be started when T-cell counts became low or after an illness with PCP. (PCP causes at least 60 percent of AIDS-related deaths, most of which could be prevented by diligently finding the best prophylaxis for each individual. The use of drugs for PCP prevention has significantly improved survival rates for PWAs.) Referrals would be immediately available if problems occurred that could not be managed in the primary care setting. When an opportunistic infection occurred and a promising experimental drug might be considered, the provider would refer the client to a drug trial, preferably a community-based one, where the experimental treatment would be given, following informed consent procedures. The primary provider would maintain involvement with the client throughout the course of the experimental treatment.

When available, this standard state-of-the-art medical care is known to prolong life and health in HIV illness. This regimen of care is available to few. Health providers who treat poor people with HIV illness see primarily people of color, women, and IVDUs. They are seeing a different spectrum of illness than is seen in economically advantaged white men. No state-of-the-art treatment standard has been established for IVDUs or women with HIV disease. To begin to create standards, the underlying medical problems that women or IVDUs face must first be addressed.

IVDUs who are actively using drugs need comprehensive care as well as immediate detoxification and treatment for addictions. Common illnesses in this group include renal and liver disease, endocarditis, cellulitis, abscesses, tuberculosis, asthma, and pulmonary disease (especially in crack smokers). IVDUs with HIV infection often die from these medical problems although they do not meet the CDC's criteria for a diagnosis of AIDS. They get sick frequently, and their immune systems are already burdened from drug use.

Women have illnesses that are not the same as those of the typical male patient. HIV-positive women often have chronic vaginitis, pelvic infections, vaginal and cervical lesions, and pulmonary infections. Unless these underlying problems are adequately treated and recurrences prevented, even state-of-the-art HIV care may fail to improve the health or extend the life of such clients.

Of course, this assumes that these persons have access to the existing medical care system, are aware of their HIV status, and want medical intervention. Many obstacles thwart this likelihood. Women, especially women with children, may have access to a provider, but this provider may be poorly trained at recognizing HIV illness in women, especially when it is asymptomatic and most amenable to treatment. IVDUs, poor people in general, prisoners, and women of color in particular have experiences of abuses within the system—for example, sterilization abuses, sexual abuses, or drug experimentation—and may be reasonably hesitant to seek health care. Poor people (who are primarily women and especially women of color) simply don't have regular access to primary health care services and therefore use public hospitals' emergency rooms. When the only option for receiving health services is to become enrolled in a clinical drug trial, it is not surprising that many such trials are not fully enrolled. Drug trials cannot become a substitute for health care services.

Do Drugs Equal Health Care?

Since virtually every drug used to fight HIV, or the concomitant opportunistic infections of AIDS, is experimental, very often one must be in a drug trial to get the drug. Yet AIDS drug trials exclude many of those infected with the virus. Women, IVDUs, hemophiliacs, children, and people of color have been systematically excluded from most experimental drug trials for AIDS therapies. Most drug trial subjects are white, well-educated, gay men living in urban areas. But this is nothing new. Drug trials have excluded most of these groups for years.[1]

The pervasive rationale used by the government to exclude women is to avoid liability for a drug's potential damage to her reproductive capacity or, if she were pregnant, to a fetus. Exclusion of other groups usually involves stereotyping them as "poor subjects" (i.e., "noncompliant") or is relegated to the difficult logistics of becoming accessible to poor people.

The AIDS movement has focused on clinical research to find drugs to treat people with AIDS, preferably a vaccine or a cure. AIDS activists are aware that this bottom-line demand fails to address many crucial health needs of all people with HIV disease, and it has particularly failed women as a strategy.

Women are excluded from drug trials explicitly and implicitly. They are required to give proof of contraception or sterilization to enroll; they are tested for pregnancy during enrollment. Trial sites do not generally consider women's special needs for child care, for appropriate transportation, and for appointments that match their needs for caring for children and other family members.

Hundreds of new drugs are tested for use in HIV illness every month. The government controls how this takes place. The agency in charge of drug testing is the Food and Drug Administration (FDA). The National Institute of Allergy and Infectious Diseases (NIAID) oversees the AIDS treatment program through its AIDS program office and by sponsoring AIDS Clinical Trial Groups (ACTGs) or by receiving applications from others (usually drug companies) who want to try a new drug out after FDA approval.

ACTGs are located at 35 hospitals around the country. In order to test a new drug, a detailed plan must be written (called a protocol) and presented to the FDA. The drug goes through several steps of approval: from test tube to animal testing to human subject testing for safety and finally efficacy (usefulness, successfulness). This process takes too long for PWAs. Activists have organized primarily around getting promising drugs into people's bodies faster. The only anti-HIV drug currently approved by the FDA for AIDS treatment is AZT.

The types of drugs currently being investigated include three categories: (1) antivirals, which have some activity against HIV; (2) immunomodulators, which enhance the immune system in some way; and (3) drugs that treat and/or prevent HIV-specific illnesses such as opportunistic infections or neoplasms.

The percentage of women enrolled in ACTG drug trials in August 1988 was about 5 percent. The percentage of people of color at the same time was 17 percent as compared to 25 percent in the national population. Underenrollment in existing trials means there are thousands of unfilled slots. Lack of enrollment of women in drug trials may be due to lack of recruitment, deliberate exclusion, or failure to meet specific needs such as child care or transportation. Of the 200 women included in drug trials in 1988, 72 percent were enrolled in AZT trials, a drug they could have gotten without entering a trial. Something is obviously wrong with this picture.

A review of trials as published by the American Foundation for AIDS Research (AmFAR) reveals that at the end of 1989 there are still blind placebo trials for adults and children (trials in which an inert substance is given to some of the trial participants without their knowledge), trials that exclude women, and trials that require proof of infertility. Various trial protocols exclude enrollees due to various factors that include active drug use, past drug use, inability to care for oneself, chronic herpes infection, use of alcohol, being pregnant, and being unable to read and write English. Some exclusions may be necessary to run drug trials; others are blatantly discriminatory.

Investigational Drugs

Some drugs present special questions for women. Hormonelike drugs will undoubtedly affect women differently. Many drugs cross the placenta, and few drugs are considered safe for a fetus, especially in the first trimester. Often the fact that a woman is capable of pregnancy excludes her from getting medications she needs or wants, regardless of her intentions regarding a present or future pregnancy.

The following drugs are all in some phase of drug testing and are worthy of mention for anyone who is considering treatment options. Most cannot be prescribed by a doctor except with approval from the FDA (called compassionate use or investigational new drug use). The saga of which drugs have been moved along rapidly in the testing process is not parallel to those that are the most promising or the least toxic.

Aerosolized pentamidine: an inhalant used to prevent episodes of PCP with little absorption from the lungs into the rest of the body. It is currently approved for use as a prophylaxis in adults. Its side effects are cough or bronchospasm during treatment. It cannot stop the pneumocystis carinii organism from causing infection in other areas of the body.

Alpha-interferon: an expensive drug used to treat Kaposi's sarcoma (KS) that may also have antiviral activity. It is given by daily injection, which can be done at home by the individual (like taking insulin shots). It often causes persistent flu-like symptoms.

Amphotericin-B: a standard antifungal medication given intravenously that is used to treat cryptoccal meningitis. It can damage the kidneys and often causes unpleasant side effects such as vomiting, fever, or chills.

Ampligen: a drug that may have both immunomodulator and antiviral activity. Early trials may have been flawed because the drug was found to lose potency in the plastic bottles it was stored in. New trials will have to be developed using nonabsorbent containers.

AZT: an antiviral drug that received FDA approval before completion of testing. It has been the subject of much controversy regarding its high cost, efficacy, and safety. It was not studied in women before FDA approval. Animal studies that reveal female reproductive cancers in mice and rats were released late in 1989. AZT was originally used in high doses associated with high toxicity and loss of effectiveness after 6 to 18 months. Fewer side effects are associated with lower-dose regimens, but efficacy is not established at lower doses. Therapies such as AZT should not be allowed to cause more medical problems than they solve, and frequent high-quality monitoring is essential. AZT is often discontinued due to side effects. It can cause severe anemia that can require blood transfusions. It may be used with other drug treatments, but, when an opportunistic infection occurs, treatment with an appropriate drug is probably more important than continuing on AZT if both drugs cannot be taken.

Bactrim (also called Septra): a well-known, standard combination antibiotic that is a good treatment for PCP as well as a prophylactic medication for PCP. It cannot be used by someone who is allergic to sulfa, and for unknown reasons many PWAs cannot tolerate this drug and develop fever or rash. PCP is the cause of death in at least 60 percent of AIDS deaths. Most of these deaths should be preventable by diligently finding the best prophylaxis for each individual. The use of drugs for PCP prevention has significantly improved survival for PWAs and should be considered a crucial part of treatment. This drug probably should be used for PCP prophylaxis in children, although it is not presently approved for such usage.

Bovine milk immune globulin: used in the treatment of diarrhea caused by cryptosporidiosis.

Compound Q (trichosanthin): a Chinese root that has shown significant antiviral activity. It has a long history of use as an abortifacient in China. It has proven to be toxic at some dosages and in some forms. The implications of its use in women and its effect on female reproductive organs need to be explored.

Dextran sulfate: an antiviral drug that inhibits HIV in the test tube, and has been used safely for 25 years in Japan for treating elevated lipids. It has been delayed in testing in the United States; meanwhile, an underground supply has been coming into this country from Japan. It may not be as effective taken orally and needs to be tested as an IV drug.

ddI (dideoxyinosine): an antiviral drug that is not as potent as AZT in inhibiting HIV in the test tube, but is considered to be less toxic. Its side effects include liver damage and nerve damage, especially to the feet.

DHEA (dehydroepiandrosterone): a testosterone-like chemical found naturally in women and men. Its natural occurrence in the body appears to be decreased in HIV infection. It may also have antiviral activity. It has been used in Italy and Japan to treat depression. Some trials have excluded women, which is common with hormonelike drugs.

DHPG (ganciclovir): an antiviral drug given intravenously for CMV retinitis (which can cause blindness). It can cause bone marrow suppression.

EPO (erythropoietin): a naturally occurring chemical found in humans that stimulates red blood cell production. Used to combat the anemia caused by AZT.

Fluconazole: an antifungal medication that appears to be effective for several fungal infections (such as cryptococcal meningitis), and is less toxic than the standard treatment, amphotericin-B.

Foscarnet: an antiviral that is active against herpes viruses including cytomegalovirus (CMV) and shows some anti-HIV activity. It may be less toxic than DHPG as a treatment for CMV infections.

GM-CSF (granulocyte-macrophage colony stimulating factor): an enzyme that stimulates production of these two types of white blood cells, and may thereby improve immune function.

Hypericin (an extract of the herb St. John's wort): an herbal medication that may have antiviral activity. It has been used extensively outside of formal drug trials because it is available by herbal distributors. More formal study is needed.

Imreg-1: derived from human blood, may have immunomodulator activity.

Lentinan: a mushroom extract that may have immune-boosting qualities.

Megace: a progestin-like hormone used in the treatment of breast cancer that may counter weight loss in PWAs.

Passive immunotherapy: a technique of filtering blood of asymptomatic HIV-positive donors to use for patients with AIDS to boost immune function by supplying doses of HIV antibodies.

Peptide T: a laboratory-made peptide (piece of a protein molecule) that is believed to inhibit the binding of HIV to the T-cells. It is considered fairly nontoxic.

Trimetrexate: another still-experimental treatment for PCP that needs further study.

Alternative and Holistic Treatments

In addition to the state-of-the-art treatment and experimental drugs for HIV illness, a spectrum of alternative therapies exists. These alternatives often embrace a holistic philosophy and stress the importance of a non-Western medical regimen alongside a nutritional approach; an exercise program; a physical modality such as traditional massage, shiatsu massage, or chiropractic adjustments; and specific stress reduction measures such as yoga, tai chi, exercise, and meditation.

The medical regimen may utilize traditional Chinese medicine (e.g., acupuncture, herbs), homeopathy, or Ayurvedic medicine. Some nutritional approaches emphasize herbal supplements and vitamins, and diets such as macrobiotics also may be viewed as a healing method.

Traditional Chinese medicine is a medical art that has been used for at least 5,000 years. It employs techniques such as acupuncture, herbs, cups (for creating suction, especially for lung expansion), heat (moxibustion), and massage. Acupuncture is used to treat illness, improve body functions, enhance energy, and as a form of nondrug anesthesia. It is also an effective nondrug treatment for detoxification of addictive chemicals, including alcohol, heroin, cocaine, and tobacco. Lincoln Hospital, a public hospital in New York City, runs a successful acupuncture clinic for drug detoxification that treats 200 to 300 patients daily. This program has also shown that acupuncture is beneficial to PWAs in terms of symptom relief as well as improvement in markers such as T-cells.

Homeopathy is a medical system that differs significantly from Western (allopathic) medicine. It was developed by a German doctor in the 1800s. It stresses using and amplifying the body's own responses instead of opposing them. Some homeopathic physicians have strategies for treatment of HIV disease that they feel are promising. These approaches have generally been disparaged by Western medical experts as unscientific. Alternative practitioners are often not eligible for insurance or Medicaid reimbursement and, being out of the mainstream, are often invisible. Until funding for exploration of all modes of treatment is undertaken, some of these promising methods will continue to exist only outside of the health care system, unavailable and unaffordable to those who might benefit from them.

Demands: A Women's Treatment Agenda

We need primary, universal health care for all people, including women and children, at all stages of HIV infection, that incorporates all of the following:

- Treatment facilities that meet all of women's needs, including transportation, child care, substance-use detoxification programs, psychological support services, peer group support, safe sex education, and nutritional counseling.
- Adequate, on-site comprehensive gynecological and obstetrical services.
- Access to experimental drugs at the site where health care is received.
- Comprehensive information and informed consent, so each woman can make her own best decision regarding experimental drugs and treatments.

We need a research agenda that incorporates women's issues and includes

- Comprehensive research into the unique aspects, natural course, and progression of HIV illness in women and children.
- Research into the effects of new drugs on women's and children's bodies, with an emphasis on the effects on women's reproductive systems.
- Research on the use of new drugs during pregnancy and their effect on both women and fetuses.
- Research into alternative, holistic models of treatment, as they affect women and children.

We need policies that promote wellness and choice in our lives as women with HIV illness, including

- No directed counseling about HIV-antibody testing, pregnancy, or medical therapies. Women need information and must be allowed and encouraged to make our own decisions.
- No coercive sterilizations, abortions, or other reproductive imperatives. Full spectrum of medical services must include obstetrics, gynecology, and abortion.
- Informed consent for experimental drugs and treatment that is specific to women.
- Government agencies, including Institutional Review Boards that oversee drug protocols, must be charged with the responsibility to determine how women will be included in all approved drug trials.
- No risk of loss of child custody due to HIV illness.
- Services such as child care, home health care, and home maintenance must be part of the comprehensive health services available to women with AIDS and HIV illness.[2]

Acknowledgments

Thanks to Deb Levine for contributions to this chapter.

Notes

1. ACT UP/New York, *FDA Action Handbook* (New York City: ACT UP, September 1988, unpublished). Available from ACT UP/NY.
2. Information for this chapter was derived from many sources. Of particular usefulness and interest are the following (please see Resources for how to contact these organizations and for more treatment resources):
   - ACT UP/NY, "AIDS Drugs Now," May 1989.
   - ACT UP/NY, "Alternative and Holistic Subcommittee Teach-In Handbook," April 1989.
   - ACT UP/NY, "Treatment and Data Digest" (weekly).
   - *AIDS Treatment News,* available from John S. James, P.O. Box 411256, San Francisco, CA 94141 (biweekly).
   - *AIDS Treatment Registry,* available from ATR.
   - Callen, Michael, ed., *Surviving and Thriving with AIDS: Collected Wisdom,* Vols. 1 (1987) and 2 (1989), (New York: PWA Coalition).
   - *Experimental Treatment Directory,* available from The American Foundation for AIDS Research
   - *Notes from the Underground,* available from PWA Health Group, 31 W. 26th St., New York, NY 10010, 212/532-0280.
   - *PWA Coalition Newsline,* available from PWA Coalition.
   - *The Body Positive: A Magazine about HIV,* available from Body Positive of New York.

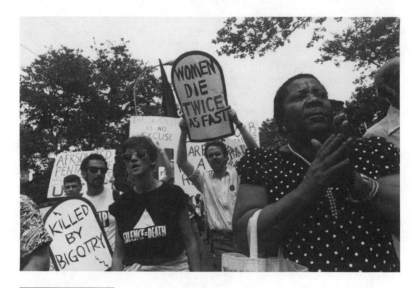

ACT UP joined with People's Alliance for Community Action, a Brooklyn-based health advocacy group, to protest the deplorable conditions at Kings County Hospital in summer 1989.

Photo by T. L. Litt

Race, Women, and AIDS: Introduction

MARION BANZHAF

Women of color account for 73 percent of women with AIDS in the United States.[1] This statistic cannot be viewed in a vacuum. It reflects the racism permeating all aspects of our society. If you want to fight racism, you have to recognize it. The extent to which white people oppose racism will to a large extent determine how effective they will be in advocating for *all* people with AIDS. Supporting universal access to health care, eliminating the disparity in life spans following an AIDS diagnosis, opposing unethical experimentation, and addressing homelessness and other survival issues are all part of dealing with the entire scope of the AIDS epidemic.

The following essays contain similar themes that are at the heart of addressing issues of race and culture. The common messages highlight the need for access to increased funding, respect for different cultural approaches, and the recognition that the affected communities themselves are best equipped to develop educational and prevention materials that are culturally appropriate.

AIDS is only the most recent health crisis to attack people of color. A common adage in the Black community is, "when white people get a cold, Black people get pneumonia."[2] Diabetes, cancer, and heart disease all strike people of color at greater rates than white people. Twenty-seven percent of Hispanics and 19.3 percent of Black people have no health insurance, compared to 12.4 percent of white people.[3] AIDS is currently the leading cause of death in women between the ages of 25 and 34 in New York City. For women of color, AIDS has genocidal ramifications. Along with infant mortality rates twice as high as those for white women, the disproportionate number of women of color affected by AIDS could mean the decimation of whole communities. Equal access to treatment and changing the entire health care system so that people's immune systems are better fortified from childhood into adulthood must become priority demands for the AIDS activist movement.

The barriers to change are great. The United States has historically enacted policies of health care discrimination and outright genocide. When the country was first colonized, it was giving smallpox-infested blankets to Native Americans. In the 1950s, under Operation Bootstrap in Puerto Rico, it was conducting massive sterilizations of women. In the 1960s, when revolutionary groups such as the Black Panthers and the Young Lords were trying to organize, there was a sudden accessibility of heroin in Black and Puerto Rican communities. Today such discriminatory policies are closing city hospitals, cutting Medicaid funds, denying funds to expand drug treatment programs, withholding treatment for AIDS based on inability to pay, and, as a result, allowing poor people of color with AIDS to die.

Changing governmental and social policies requires joint work among AIDS activists. Building coalitions and working together isn't easy. Often, everyone has to suspend some issues to be able to work together and build a basis of respect. As Bernice Johnson Reagon has said about coalition politics, "I feel as if I'm gonna keel over any minute and die. That is often what it feels like if you're really doing coalition work. Most of the time you feel threatened to the core and if you don't, you're not really doing no coalescing."[4] We all bring our histories with us.

People of color don't need "charity activists." Coalition efforts are most successful when everyone is fighting in their own interest for a common goal. What works best is the recognition that everyone fighting together, in coalition, in alliance, or separately with communication, can create a stronger base that has more potential to win change than if we fight separately.

ACT UP remains mostly a white, male group. As mostly white women, we have had to fight for our visibility, as have the people of color in the organization. We women have argued with the men that it is their responsibility to listen to us and to take up issues of sexism. As well, we think it is the responsibility of white people to oppose racism and to act on issues raised by people of color.

The following essays explore issues of AIDS and racism in various communities. For further reading, *Our Lives in the Balance: U.S. Women of Color and the AIDS Epidemic,* coedited by Alma Crawford, Val Kanuha, Aleah Long, Veneita Porter, Dr. Helen Rodriguez, and Beverly Smith and published by Kitchen Table:

Women of Color Press in 1991, and *The Black Women's Health Book: Speaking for Ourselves,* edited by Evelyn C. White and published by Seal Press, are essential sources for further understanding issues about women of color and AIDS.

Acknowledgments

Special thanks to Dr. Iris Davis, Dr. Yannick Durand, Suki Ports, and Sunny Rumsey for the time, knowledge, and support they lent to this project. Judith Walker contributed to this section.

Notes

1. Centers for Disease Control, *HIV/AIDS Surveillance Report,* January 1990, pp. 1-16.
2. Evelynn Hammonds, "Race, Sex, AIDS: The Construction of 'Other'," *Radical America,* Vol. 20, no. 6, November-December 1986.
3. Maxine Wolfe, original statistical comparison, *The ACT UP Women's Caucus Women and AIDS Handbook* (New York, NY: ACT UP, original edition, March 1989), p. 9A.
4. Bernice Johnson Reagon, "Coalition Politics: Turning the Century," in *Home Girls: A Black Feminist Anthology,* Barbara Smith, editor (Latham, NY: Kitchen Table: Women of Color Press, 1983), p. 356.

Cultural Sensitivity in Practice

YANNICK DURAND

Overcoming a History of Powerlessness

Language is the least of the cultural problems faced by women of Caribbean descent when it comes to AIDS. For Caribbean women—that is, Haitians, Jamaicans, Hispanics, and so on—their culture does not allow them to be as assertive as the American health system *requires*. This has nothing to do with class; it's a frame of mind. In some of these countries, the service does not even exist.

As a native of Haiti, I can speak best of that country. Haiti lacks doctors and medical facilities, or, if they exist, they don't even have the basics, like cotton balls and syringes. For example, when people go to a hospital they have to buy medicines outside. So Haitians in the United States do not realize, first, that the service exists, and second, that it's theirs. Therefore, at the Brooklyn AIDS Task Force (BATF) we cannot offer education only about HIV and HIV prevention: we also have to teach about the health system itself and how it works. Women need this more than men do because most of the time they have lower-paying jobs; they have less direct contact with the system; they're also more likely to have the lowest literacy level (if anyone in the family goes to school, it won't be the woman). Actually, what it would take is for people to become part of the community, even before addressing AIDS or health care. At BATF, we deal with all our clients' needs, not just AIDS issues.

A lot of Third World people don't accept the buddy system, for example, because they're suspicious of outsiders intruding on their privacy and might think they would want to control them. They're used to being controlled; resignation is part of our background, our luggage. Bias is an important issue for our clients. At BATF, we don't tell people what to do; we give them information and try to empower them to make their own decision. We work with them so that they can build up their self-esteem. (We prefer to use that word; the concept of empowerment is a bit too political and can therefore be viewed by some as threatening, but in fact it comes to the same thing.) It helps that our staff represents various cultures, sexual orientations, and both genders.

Another problem in getting Haitians to accept the concept of AIDS prevention is their inner belief system. The main religions in Haiti are voodoo and Catholicism. Catholicism teaches you resignation and guilt, and in voodoo you can be harmed by someone who isn't present, who isn't even real. Haitians who are used to voodoo have a hard time taking responsibility for their health in any way. I've often heard of HIV diseases as sent to people as a curse. Once a woman told me that gay men had received AIDS as a punishment from God; I replied, "Then lesbians must be God's chosen group since they seem to be the least affected." That seemed to make her think.

Much of what I'm saying applies mainly to Haitian adults. The kids are much more Americanized through school, where they make friends from other cultures. This causes a conflict of cultures at home, but Haitians are very proud of their children's ability to make it here. It's very rare for a Haitian child not to finish high school. Education is considered a weapon for escaping from low socioeconomic status. It's too soon to say how these aspects of Haitian culture will persist over time—Haitians are still new in America. (They started coming in the late 1950s and early 1960s, when Duvalier came to power.)

Sexual Attitudes

As far as sex is concerned, people do it, but they don't talk about it. It's considered normal for Haitian men to sleep with many women, but divorce is not common in this culture. Gender roles are very strong. The man is perceived to be sensual, to have sexual needs, and the woman to have feelings. He takes the initiative and enjoys sex, while she puts up with it. Because the traditional roles are so rigid, men will talk to men about sex, and women will talk to women, but they won't talk to each other. (See *Se Met Ko,* a Haitian educational video about AIDS, by Patricia Benoit.) So AIDS educators and service providers need to respect that inner structure whether they agree with it or not.

Some Haitian women can't even say out loud that they sleep with their own husbands. Consequently, many Haitian children have never seen their parents physically touch each other.

Teenage girls are expected to marry early—by age 25 at the latest—but not to date. When they marry, they're supposed to be virgins. Probably they *don't* sleep around much. As for the kids, they generally go to Catholic schools, where there's not much open talk about AIDS.

According to most Haitians, this is the only culture in the world in which homosexuality does not exist! Of course it exists. But there is absolute denial. It is considered a shame for the whole family if one member is gay. This attitude has even hardened as a result of AIDS. Haitians will see only homosexuality in an openly gay person; they won't hear anything else he or she says. It would be crazy for gay men to come talk to Haitians about AIDS only from a gay perspective. Crazy! Because the Haitians won't hear the information itself but only as it is connected to the sexual orientation of the speaker, and therefore not valid for them. This denial has made Haitians extremely resistant to hearing about AIDS and dealing with it in their own community.

What does all this mean for AIDS education? It means a big part of our job is getting people used to hearing and saying words like "condom" and "intercourse." We're trying to make these words part of people's everyday lives. But it can't be done by force; our expectations must be realistic. It can be a big victory just to get a young man to accept a condom at a health fair. If a woman insists that her child isn't "doing anything wrong," that is, having sex, we don't insist that she face facts. We say, "Of course not, but your neighbor's child might be," and build on her concern for her neighbors.

Outreach

You'd be amazed how many people live in New York for years without knowing how to get out of their neighborhoods. This is true of a good half of the Haitian population (and this is certainly not limited to Haitians; there's a whole non-middle-class America that's passive because it doesn't realize the power it can acquire through knowledge). So at BATF, we find ways (we have to) to get to them.

To have an impact on the Haitian community (as in any culture), you have to go to the women. They're the ones who carry on the traditions; they're the ones who are active in the church and the parents' associations. And you have to go to the children. For immigrants who are parents, their kids are their link with the system; the kids are the ones coming home with information. Also, kids have less accumulated social prejudice than adults, and fewer sexual hangups. And they're obviously the best outreach workers for getting to other kids.

We go everywhere, from the church to block parties, from the parents' association to the last-born child's baptism—not just into a mythic "community." We train leaders from the community to educate their own. For example, we can't get into Catholic schools, so we go to youth centers or Y's nearby and make friends with a few kids. We train them and reward them with T-shirts, gym bags, pens...they go back to school and talk to their friends. Even if we don't reach every kid directly, the ones trained become peer educators.

Methods of HIV/AIDS Education

Sex is not just the main, but really is the only route of transmission for HIV among Haitians. I'd say drug use, if there is any, is not a major issue. Haitians are not into substances; that's not our way of getting away from reality. So in doing AIDS education for this group we focus on sexual transmission.

We've found one of the most powerful motives for both women and men to use condoms is not to save their own lives, but to stay around for their children. They'll protect themselves for the sake of their kids. Or because their extended family, their community, needs them. You see, in Western civilization, people learn to do things for themselves; they say "I" a lot, an "I" that seems to be an isolated entity. In other cultures, like in Haiti, people learn to do for others. They tend to say "we," or "I" as part of "we." They're individuals within a group. If you tell Haitians that a condom can save their life, they shrug. Often for these people life is already so dangerous; in their homeland and here in their neighborhoods, they face poverty, racism, drugs, crime, you name it. Also, women often depend on men for social status, financial support, self-esteem—they're afraid they'll lose their men if they make them wear condoms (which equals taking away their virility). So getting people used to condoms is a long and very difficult process.

Literature is not all that important a tool for this population. The type of work they usually do is physically exhausting: factory work, home care, housework, and so on. They don't have the time or the energy to read. At BATF, we work with visual tools like videos. We make practical things like calendars, T-shirts, pens; we have a key chain on a little box for condoms with the motto "In Condom I Trust." And we use word of mouth—we do a lot of presentations to different community groups and we table all over the place.

As far as language is concerned, it's a rather difficult choice. Some people speak Creole, others French. We try to offer them their choice.

When you do AIDS education with Haitians, you have to get personal. They want to know all about you, your mother, your father.

You can talk for hours before you touch the topic of AIDS! To bring it up too directly would defeat the purpose.

It just doesn't work to bring Haitians, or for that matter most non-middle-class people, together just to talk about AIDS. At BATF, we have a lot of activity groups. For women, there might be groups for sewing, knitting, or skill building. For teenagers, we have pizza parties, drawing groups, and so on. AIDS information is conveyed, but it's not the main focus. People love our activity groups who would never go to an AIDS program, but they end up very well informed about AIDS.

I'm focusing on education because that's my job, but there must also be culturally sensitive ways of providing services to PWAs. For example, the support groups used successfully by the organizations that serve gay white men don't really work for people who are not middle class and therefore not accustomed to talking about themselves and their feelings for an hour in front of other people. Instead, when we want to bring PWAs or HIV positives together, we have nutrition groups or hold housing workshops in which they focus on something practical, not on themselves. Often these groups end up going to the movies together, having parties, and so on. They are support groups, but they're not only that, and that's not what they're called. To come back to the example of the buddy system, it too is based on a middle-class concept, volunteerism. If you're struggling to make ends meet, you don't have time to be a buddy. One can't just import middle-class volunteers, one needs also to train them to work respectfully with people of a totally different background.

Recommendations

The bureaucracy needs drastically to streamline the way it gives out money. The amount of time and paperwork required from small service organizations is crazy and a waste of time when you consider the urgency of needs of the communities to be served.

All organizations providing AIDS services should have multicultural staffs in order to reach a broader spectrum of the targeted populations and to develop effective educational materials for these groups. The process of developing materials should be (1) to find out from the target population what they feel is needed and in what form, (2) to develop materials jointly with the target population, and (3) to test the materials with the target population before distribution. You can't be sitting in a carpeted office in mid-Manhattan and conceptualize what's needed in Bed-Stuy.

There has to be an attitude of mutual respect and willingness to learn from each other among the different cultural and ethnic groups that have been suddenly thrown together by the AIDS epidemic. Obviously exploitation is not pleasant. What's happening now is that the big established AIDS groups are going to the small ones under the pretext of working together and learning about "minority outreach." In practice, they end up ripping off their ideas and getting big grants based on their longer track records and their experience with the funding establishment. Then the smaller groups don't have the money to service their own communities, including Haitians, for example, which they *do* know how to work with. People have to learn that *nobody* has a monopoly on this epidemic.

More education has to be targeted to specific cultural and ethnic groups. For example, with all the AIDS education that's going on, Haitians are still being ignored; they seem to be invisible in New York. This is a bunch of people that is totally left out by the experts, the AIDS educators. Actually this is not too smart of the experts. Unless we reach out to all ethnic groups, we can't expect to have long-term results.

About the Author

Yannick Durand holds a Ph.D. and works with the Brooklyn AIDS Task Force. This essay is based on an interview with Judith Walker.

First There Was Smallpox

CHARON ASETOYER

In 1985, a group of Native Americans living on or near the Yankton Sioux Reservation in South Dakota formed the Native American Community Board to address pertinent issues of health, education, land and water rights, and economic development of Native American people. The first NACB project developed was "Women, Children, and Alcohol," a fetal alcohol syndrome program. It was through the Women, Children, and Alcohol program that we were able to define the direction of our work. In February 1988, the Native American Community Board opened the first Native American Women's Health Education Resource Center located on a reservation in the United States. It is based in Lake Andes, South Dakota, on the Yankton Sioux Reservation.

In June 1988, I went to a conference in Washington, D.C., sponsored by the National Women's Health Network and attended by approximately 60 of the country's most active health feminists. Many health advocates working in the front lines of the AIDS crisis attended this conference, and it was there that I became very involved in learning more about people of color and AIDS. This past spring (1989), I attended a meeting in New York City at the Center for Constitutional Rights (CCR) concerning people of color and AIDS.

As a Native American woman, I have had very mixed feelings about many issues surrounding the AIDS crisis. Often I find myself amidst confrontation among both Native Americans and non-Native Americans due to the complexity of the issue. The more involved I got, the clearer it became that there was a need for the facts to be documented.

AIDS is a complex issue for all cultures, but even more so for Native Americans. AIDS has now reached even the most remotely located Native American community. Though Native Americans have survived the purposeful introduction of smallpox, tuberculosis, and many other viruses into our culture by the U.S. government, AIDS presents new dangers. There are an estimated 1.4 million Native Americans both on and off reservations in the United States. The census identifies 278 reservations and 209 Alaskan native villages. Thirty-seven percent of the population lives inside identified Indian areas as defined by the census, such as reservations and villages.

Native American people are presently in all risk groups and engage in high-risk behavior. There's often an unwillingness on the part of the administrators working with Native Americans and among Native Americans ourselves to recognize the prevalence of homosexual and bisexual behavior in our communities. Also, there is a belief that IV drug use is uncommon, and that is untrue...it's very common in urban population areas. Native Americans have additional health problems which may add to the transmission of the HIV virus, including high rates of sexually transmitted diseases and alcoholism. On reservation-based communities, alcoholism is one of the main high-risk behavior factors.

Native Americans are in the lowest economic bracket, are less educated, die younger, suffer more health problems and substance abuse, and go to prisons more often than many other populations. Native Americans have far inferior access to health care, and greater incidence of poor diets, unemployment, communicable diseases, respiratory infections, accidents, homicides, and suicides than the population as a whole.

The poor health of Native Americans may speed the development of AIDS in an HIV-infected individual. Lack of access to advanced health care and technology, and the means to pay for it, will hasten death with the onset of opportunistic diseases. Health care for Native Americans is of lower quality and a greater distance from our homes than it is for the general population. It's not uncommon to have to travel 100-150 miles just to get to the clinic or the Indian Health Service (IHS) hospital. Native American people with AIDS are confronted with problems similar to non-Indian people with AIDS but lack many of the support services, legal guidance, and treatment options available to middle-class, white, urban residents.

Women suffer disproportionately in the Native American community. They are more often the victims of abuse, and, as the sole family providers, are the least economically advantaged of any group in the country. Native American women may be at risk of infection with the HIV virus because of the prevalence of bisexual and non-monogamous behavior among Native American men and the lack of safe sex awareness and behavior.

Confidentiality for AIDS testing and treatment is just about nonexistent in small communities, especially in the IHS hospitals. Many states do not offer anonymous testing, including South Dakota, North Dakota, Iowa, Nebraska, Minnesota. These are all of the states that surround the Aberdeen area office of the Indian Health Service, which provides services to our community.

Calls for mandatory testing are ill-advised, but that attitude does exist in our community. Many people call for mandatory testing without understanding the full legal conflict. People think that they will get this information so they'll know whether their neighbor is HIV positive or not, and don't understand the process or the implications of mandatory testing. They think this information will be open to John Doe Public and that's incorrect.

We're also dealing with the issue of blind testing. The Centers for Disease Control (CDC) and the IHS have been doing a blind study of HIV testing on Native Americans nationwide. This became an issue during the Native American caucus at the 1987 National Minority AIDS Conference in Washington, D.C. I brought it to the attention of the caucus that the CDC and the IHS were about to launch a blind testing campaign. E.Y. Hooper, an official among the higher echelons of the IHS and one of the people in charge of addressing the AIDS epidemic among Native American populations (assigned by the IHS), informed us that there would be blind testing. He basically said the study was needed to get appropriate funding through Congress for Native Americans. Since when is blind testing a prerequisite for major funding? You don't put people on hold until you calculate your facts and statistics.

At the 1989 Minority AIDS Conference, the Native American caucus again brought up the issue of blind testing. We were informed by the CDC and the IHS' Hooper that just about 50 percent of the tribes in the United States had undergone blind testing.

One of the groups that have been targeted for blind testing is pregnant women who are receiving prenatal care. How dare they not inform a pregnant woman that she may be HIV positive! Testing pregnant women presents a whole array of problems. To fulfill its responsibility as the primary health care provider for Native Americans, the IHS would have to provide a service that it does not provide—giving the woman the option of terminating her pregnancy if she felt her health might be jeopardized. Another group of people who are included in the blind study is people being treated for sexually transmitted diseases (STDs). People being treated for STDs need to know their test results and receive safe-sex information so they do not go back into the community and spread the virus. Another study group is people in alcohol and drug treatment. They too need to know if they are HIV positive and how they might constructively confront the risks they face.

In Oklahoma, the IHS has been caught doing blind testing by taking blood at health fairs under the auspices of providing a blood cholesterol count. But the blood is not taken from a finger prick, but from the arm, and they give you a notice saying that you are participating in a blind study. If you refuse to participate in the study, they don't even take your blood for the cholesterol count. So they aren't really interested in the cholesterol count; they're interested only in the results for HIV.

As of 1989, there were approximately 150 cases of AIDS reported by the CDC among Native Americans. When you know that for every one case of AIDS there are projected to be 100 HIV-positive people, you've got to look at the impact that has on our population. We're looking at 1 percent and we're headed toward 2 percent of the total Native American population nationwide being infected.

IHS is still not appropriating any significant funding for education and services. In 1988, our reservation got about $1,000 from the IHS for education. That's definitely an inappropriate amount. By the time the figures come in from the blind testing study, there are going to be a lot more Native Americans infected. The IHS seems to think that we can just put this epidemic on hold. Well, AIDS is not an on-hold disease.

About the Author

Charon Asetoyer is Executive Director of the Native American Women's Health Education Resource Center. She is also a member of the advisory board of the Center for Constitutional Rights' Education and Legal Advisory Project for Women and People of Color.

No Names and No Pictures

IRIS DAVIS

Like so many of the women we treated from our surrounding community, Sandy could not cope with being at risk for HIV or having HIV disease. Although her husband had died recently from AIDS, she could not envision that the destruction of her family came about due to a past and infrequent behavior. Sandy's issues were stability, loyalty, family, and raising children—certainly not behavior in her husband of ten years that she had never seen or heard about. The anger in her voice was sincere and directed toward those who put her husband in the context of a drug addict. She had knowledge of drug addicts; her neighborhood was one where the balance was delicate and difficult to maintain. The "labeling" was a recurrent theme at our clinic. Somehow, the spectrum of disease or behavior or life was not a possibility for the worlds our patients inhabited. Other people saw them in stark and somber colors, not muted or in hues varying as individuals or even as groups.

At times, the waiting room seemed to be a mini-United Nations. Children racing across the floor, Muslim women sitting in their statuesque enrobements, Hispanic women speaking to one another in one language, although from four different countries, Haitians, African-Americans, Russian Jews from Bensonhurst—a panoply of cultures connected by a virus and by fear. Hope was not as catching, but it bounced in and out also.

There were too few small, community-based, publicly funded clinics like our HIV family care center. Our center was always disquietingly "unique" due to the "populations" we attracted—just like the individuals from the same populations that staffed the clinic. Those populations could have been more statistics for New York City—80 percent IVDU and 20 percent male—to study risk behaviors. We heard other stories, of drugs used on weekends, holidays, a decade ago. We heard of changed behaviors, or hidden "secret" periods; respected images and jobs; children who were in school now; wives that had never known, never needed to know about the drug use; what would happen to their mortgages, car loans, tuition payments!

Histories and physicals are always vignettes of people's lives distilled to help the healers see what is bothering the story tellers. That was too often why they chose our clinic. They told us we cared, or did not judge, or looked like their mothers, sisters, daughters, all the women in their life. Folks varied from extremely poor, homeless, to borderline with jobs off the books, people who had worked all their lives with the wrong kind of insurance papers, to middle-income people who could not obtain HIV/AIDS care under their insurance providers. Other times they came because this was the clinic for a community that straddled common, hidden behaviors and many cultures, and this is where the hospital sent them. Sent them to the "famous" clinic, our favored clinic, where appointments were made four to six weeks away for too few providers and there were still too many walk-ins to slow down or eat lunch. The pressure from the numbers forced us to become premiere curtain pullers. We allowed little denial—it blocked treatment, safer sex, and prevention.

Stereotypes are often held by the same people that other groups think are the stereotypes. It just wasn't there. Too frequently, a job, functioning family, and community responsibilities were badges of courage that denied possibilities of HIV. It had to happen to "bad" people—or "those" people—who would have ever thought it was me?

Sandy's anger had been directed when she was in the wheel-chair that she needed due to paralyzed and spastic legs. Her meningitis would require treatment all her life. A woman who had worked since the age of 18 waited for five months for a social service system to find her a part-time housekeeper so she could continue parenting her seven- and nine-year-old children.

For five months, she lay in a hospital bed, looking at her nurses, dressed as she was dressed every day until she became ill. In the peak years of her life, she is now a shadow of herself and a widow trying to make a wholeness from the shrapnel caused by a blood-borne virus.

When she first described her wish to organize people like herself, I gave her names. When she mentioned a need to march, I called for transportation so her voice could be heard. She never called the people, and she missed the demonstration. Now we were facing one another across a tiny cramped office. Today, I could turn my chair because Sandy had shuffled into my office with a walker. Talking about a cheerleader—I only needed pompoms as she proudly navigated the hall, stylishly dressed with makeup and even a new manicure. Actually, I thought that her mood would make it easier to ask her to try the newspaper interview. In a daily paper read by millions, it would make a difference. It was a chance to dispel a little more denial. Make one more affected person a human being who wanted treatment and wanted to live.

The answer was no!

"No names."

"No."

I called the journalist.

"No pictures!"

"No."

"No names and no pictures?"

"No."

"Why not?"

"I never think about AIDS. No one knows what's wrong with me except my mother. Nobody really believes I have AIDS, and no one knows I come here."

"Sandy, who will know it's you?"

"No—You don't have AIDS and two kids."

It was weeks before we established our old relationship. We never discussed AIDS as a reality for people of color again, or what happened to women with AIDS, or what happened to children whose parents had AIDS.

I've left the clinic now, but my nurse/comrade-in-arms tells me Sandy is still a survivor, and I hear she is walking better.

About the Author

Iris L. Davis is a practicing physician.

We Have the Expertise, We Need Resources

RUTH RODRIGUEZ

Over one quarter of the persons with AIDS in New York City are Hispanic. Of the growing number of women with AIDS, one-third are Hispanic. According to the Centers for Disease Control, the incidence of AIDS among Hispanic women is over 11 times that for white women.

While these statistics demonstrate the overall picture in New York City, they do not begin to show the devastation occurring in latino neighborhoods. For example, in the Lower East Side, over 40 percent of all persons who died of AIDS were Hispanic.

What does the presence of a deadly, presently incurable disease, that can be prevented but that is fraught with superstition, fear, and social stigma, mean in the Hispanic community? It means a woman hiding in her apartment, if she's lucky enough to have housing, taking care of her sick son, who may be gay. Since homosexuality is a lifestyle that is even more strongly repudiated in the latino value system than it is in the general population, it means that the extended family will not be likely to help.

It means a woman whose husband has been using IV drugs, sometimes without her knowledge, having to care for him because he's contracted the disease, while waiting for the disease to strike her or her infant children.

It means a woman who has the disease and whose strength is failing, explaining to her children that she is going to die and preparing for their care without her. It means many, many more Hispanic women who are unnecessarily afraid to reach out to their stricken family members and neighbors, because they think casual contact will infect them; but these same women are not taking any measures to protect themselves from the real risks they face.

Hispanic culture and values are a hardy system that has survived and flourished throughout the Western hemisphere because it takes new situations and new information and adapts.

In order to weather the HIV epidemic, we must have information; but it is not enough that this information, the message for survival, be delivered in Spanish. Any Spanish-speaking person is horrified by the translation that presents English-language concepts in Spanish words. One English word does not equal another Spanish word.

Language is the mirror of culture, values, feelings, experience. Latino activists demand not only original, Spanish-language materials, but also that latinos be provided with information that taps the cultural/value codes that we respond to. Many latino young people do not read Spanish; many were never taught to read at all, but they respond to recognizably latino images. We need to see an AIDS prevention message that "speaks to us," that taps our belief system and develops new survival attitudes for the age of AIDS.

AIDS prevention education must be aimed at both men and women. Too often we have urged latina women to protect themselves by using condoms, only to be asked, "Will you speak to my husband?" Gender roles are very entrenched in our culture. AIDS does not afford us the time to address this, so we must use these roles to promote new behaviors. "Macho" is not unique to the latino culture, and the notion of a strong and dominant man is not something we are going to change overnight. We can, however, adapt the image and use that image to say it is "macho" to protect your own, because that is very much a part of latino values. We can teach our men to protect their own and make this acceptable within our community and within that gender role.

The print and electronic communications media that so readily and so creatively lend themselves to changing dress, deodorant use, and, yes, sexual attitudes and behavior, must be used to reach all our Hispanics—Spanish- and English-speaking.

And we believe that we cannot afford to rely on established AIDS-related institutions that have not been able to provide us with adequate education, preventive health care, or social services to do the job. We urge that all these institutions work in concert with the latino community, respecting our right to self-determination. Latino men and women who understand and represent our bilingual, bicultural community must be at the forefront in the war against AIDS. Only then can we be assured that this war will be fought on our behalf and not against us.

This country must commit public and private resources to a massive education campaign that will help change high-risk behaviors while creating an atmosphere of compassion and common purpose in the age of AIDS. But we must recognize that information cannot be imposed by one group on another. The only way to do this is to respect, support, and utilize the strengths, talents, and potential for change in each of this country's racial and ethnic communities.

We have been developing educational materials on a catch-as-catch-can basis. So the expertise certainly is there. What we need to create is a more formal structure that specifically addresses the many segments of the Hispanic population.

We have IV drug users, we have family members of IV drug users, we have gays, we have professionals and workers—we are part of a general population that is very much afraid but that does not readily discuss sex. I have been able to sit down and discuss sex with latino men and women, because I am latina myself.

Funding must be made available to bolster community-based AIDS prevention, education, and direct services for latinos.

We are struggling to develop service programs in poorer communities to meet the needs of people who are infected, and we are observing that many people are not coming forward to participate in these facilities because there is not a latino face or someone who can speak Spanish there.

The latino community does have people who are quite capable, but they have been providing services on a very limited basis because they don't have resources. We need more than stopgap services that are not adequately addressing our community's needs. We have to develop a strategy for the entire health crisis, including prenatal and well-baby care to address the high infant mortality rate, geriatric care for our elderly, and more low-income housing. There cannot be a commitment to addressing HIV infection without a commitment to *health*.

About the Author

Ruth Rodriguez was a founding board member and then Executive Director of the Hispanic AIDS Forum. She is currently Executive Director of Loisaida, Inc., a nonprofit organization serving youth and families in the Lower East Side of New York City.

AIDS Issues for African-American and African-Caribbean Women

SUNNY RUMSEY

In early 1988, 90 percent of AIDS cases in New York City were men and 10 percent were women. Now the numbers are 85 percent and 13 percent. The number of new cases among gay white men is decreasing slightly while the rate among Black and Hispanic men having sex with other men is still rising. Also, Hispanic women now account for more cases of sexually transmitted AIDS than Black women—they have the highest rate of infection through sexual contact in the city—but they don't realize it. They're not getting infected through casual sexual contact—most of these women are in monogamous relationships.

AIDS, on top of everything else, is breaking the back of the communities of people of color. Our women are in serious trouble. After eight years in this epidemic, the government has made little effort to communicate this emergency to Black and Latina women.

Information is not reaching these communities as fast as it reached the gay communities. There has been denial around AIDS in the African-American and African-Caribbean communities, but it comes in part from the lack of education as to how HIV will *infect* and *affect* their communities. People weren't prepared to work with the gay community in this crisis.

Homosexuality is rarely acknowledged within Black and Latino communities and this has affected their response to AIDS. People of color don't see the gay community as anything but white, since most men of color who have sex with men are bisexual and don't openly identify themselves as bi or gay within their communities. People assume most infected men of color are drug users, but actually almost half are gay or bisexual. An AIDS death in the family is a sensitive issue, and can be further complicated if the person was in the closet and the family didn't know. We must continue to reach into the community to help them understand that a man who dies of AIDS, whether he's 5-years-old or 35-years-old, is still someone's "child/baby."

Many people in our communities first heard of AIDS as germ warfare. When people of color with AIDS entered the overburdened medical system, they saw they weren't given the same level of care as their white counterparts. In addition, there was distrust of the government when people of color realized that little effort was being made to target resources to fight the epidemic in their communities. All of this combined to cause some segments of these communities to suspect the government of wanting to eliminate part of their population.

If you look at recent history you can understand why some parts of our communities would feel that way. Black people haven't forgotten that, during the 1960s, at the height of the Black Power movement, heroin suddenly became widely available on their streets; that had a crippling effect on the movement. New York is one of 11 states where, if you're caught carrying a needle, you can be arrested. If you can get locked up for possessing a needle, you're going to start sharing. The law actually set up a new behavior among IV drug users that spread the virus when AIDS came along.

There's a lot of subtle and not so subtle pressure on HIV-positive women, most of whom are women of color, to have abortions or get sterilized. Why should these women be treated any differently from white women with a family history of cancer, genetically transferable disease, chronic fatigue, multiple sclerosis, or a variety of deforming disabilities? Many diseases are transferred in utero, and the law strongly protects the rights of women with these diseases. To advocate for sterilization and abortion because of a disease that affects primarily women of color looks like racism. The rights of these women must be respected. There are tough issues here that we have to make more of an effort to examine, and we have to do it by consulting these women themselves and the organizations that come from and represent their communities.

These communities need more information and counseling on preventing AIDS through safer sex and better health care, and they have to be able to decide for themselves how to do it in a way that will work for them. The government must support this work without dictating that it follow a model developed by and for a different community. For example, it's not appropriate for safer-sex education for the African-American and African-Caribbean communities to suggest that women advance or take care of themselves at the expense of their men, or to assume that women by themselves can negotiate safer sex. Both women and men have to be targeted and taught about protection and responsibility. We have to train counselors to teach couples how to communicate complex issues better and in a non-threatening manner.

It's imperative that we deal with our adolescents and recognize that many adults who were diagnosed with AIDS in their twenties were actually infected in their teens. We need to take a serious look at the teen pregnancy, STD, and abortion rates in our communities and figure out what this means for AIDS and what our message to youth should be. There's a tremendous amount of sexual activity associated with crack, and this too has a big impact on the spread of AIDS. Crack is the drug of choice among the young.

Even though there are many life-and-death issues for the communities of color, AIDS must become a high priority or it will destroy us. On the positive side, agencies will be coming into their own in the 1990s that reflect these communities and that will take a leading role in AIDS advocacy and education for people of color. The change will come from within—it has to.

Recommendations

We need to be planning for the future—not relying on slogans like "just say no" and not just responding to crises in a reaction mode. We need to give people more alternatives to behaviors that put them at risk for AIDS.

As the epidemic shifts, the funding must follow. We will need more health care professionals, social workers, and advocates from and for the communities of color, and we will have to find ways to get people to enter these professions, which traditionally offer low salaries and awful working conditions, rather than business or the private sector. Since so many of these professionals are predominantly female, professional women's organizations and labor unions need to take this on as an issue and upgrade pay and working conditions.

We need better community education to help our communities and schools to accept PWAs and not reject them, whether they are students or colleagues.

We need more drug treatment programs that are sensitive to the needs of women, including pregnant women and mothers who would forgo treatment if their children could not continue to live with them.

The CDC needs to redefine AIDS as the disease manifests itself in women. The current definition is based on men's bodies. As a result, women are getting opportunistic infections related to HIV, and they're not getting an AIDS diagnosis. That means they don't get the financial assistance that people get with "official" AIDS. Many HIV-infected women are mothers and heads of households. We've got to get help to them.

People of color need to be in decision-making, policy-making positions in AIDS service organizations—not just support roles.

Women of color and from all different ethnic backgrounds need their own groups—most women still aren't organized to help themselves—and we need to build coalitions representing all these groups. No one group can stop this epidemic. Women's issues cut across all boundaries. There should be a multicultural national or regional group, composed of women who are tops in their fields, with at least three to five years of AIDS experiences, to look at how the epidemic is affecting us. And in these coalitions we have to listen to each other; we have to listen to all women's experiences, not just the skills of a few. We have to respect cultural and regional differences and let different solutions emerge from within different communities. We can't exploit our sisters, and we can't allow anyone else to. We have to try to turn around those who are with us for the wrong reasons—for example, because AIDS is a good career right now, or to advance some personal agenda. We *all* need to learn how to grow and expand so what we say and do is richer.

As people, each of us must start by looking at herself and asking how sensitive she is to the needs of her sisters. Any of us can potentially be infected, but all of us are clearly affected by this epidemic—all of us must be involved in fighting together to end it.

About the Author

Sunny Rumsey, of African-Caribbean and Native American descent, has been an AIDS activist and professional since 1985. A former director of the New York City Department of Health Community AIDS Education Program (one of the largest multicultural AIDS education programs in the United States), she is a noted spokesperson on the impact of AIDS on people of color. She is Director of Ecumenical Services for the Black Leadership Commission on AIDS. Based on an interview with Judith Walker.

Many Cultures, Many Approaches

with MARION BANZHAF

The Myth of Asian/Pacific Islanders as a Monolithic Group

The fact that there are many Asian and Pacific Island cultures is often overlooked. Each one can't be reached the same way or in the same language. The lack of understanding is part of a U.S. attitude toward peoples of other nations. Europeans are known by their country of origin—French or German—but Asians are all the same: Asians. We don't assume all Europeans are the same, and most Americans know there are different languages such as French, Dutch, Swedish, or Greek. That's not the same with Asians. When Asians are all lumped together, there are major problems in AIDS prevention, education, and treatment.

The same mind-set says there could be one kind of education for Asians, whose origins are from over 20 nations. When you bring up 32 possible dialects, people gasp and say it'd be too expensive. Even when educational materials are printed in Spanish, it's clear that Chicanas/Mexicanas are not happy with translations done primarily for Puerto Ricans or East Coast Spanish-speaking people. When education of the public depends on language and on understanding, particularly subtle nuances, and understanding doesn't exist, there's trouble.

Asians and Pacific Islanders represent more than 32 languages and dialects—even within the same nations, as seen clearly in the Philippine Islands and China. To assume someone from one Asian background can interact with or teach sensitively someone from another Asian background is incorrect.

The whole myth of this ethnic group as one monolithic group, Asians, must be challenged. The stereotypes are that Asians are not low income, are ambitious, and are well educated. But none of that applies to immigrants. If they don't speak English, they are not going

Many Cultures, Many Approaches 107

to understand an AIDS brochure. Moreover, they aren't going to understand the AIDS crisis and seek information in their own language.

"Other" = Racism

A major problem in fighting AIDS among Asians and Pacific Islanders is the tendency to discount Asian women because the numbers are still relatively low. In the United States, there are 66 women (compared to 682 men and 9 children) of Asian and Pacific Islander descent with CDC-defined AIDS (as of January 1990). However, the statistics are not broken down by year or generation of immigration to the United States. In California, cases were highest among Filipinos, then, in descending order, Japanese, Vietnamese, and Chinese. In New York City, the highest number of cases was also among Filipinos, then Chinese, Japanese, and Thai. But the statistics are still sketchy. The country of origin could be identified either by the doctor or by the patient. But one of the main problems is identification in the first place.

Because statistics are not given by all government departments of health in the same way, it is difficult to pinpoint age and country of ethnic origin. The Centers for Disease Control started to separate Asian and Pacific Islanders from Native Americans in 1988, after Asian activists identified the inadequacy of the "other" category. But in New York state, Asians, Pacific Islanders, Native Americans, and Native Alaskans are still all lumped together as "other." New York state does not even footnote the statistics, so someone not familiar with what "other" means would not know that this alludes to Asians and Native Americans. This is inherently racist. New York City puts Asians and Native Americans together, making it difficult for anyone to determine which people are in which specific age or risk category.

The peak ages of Asian women with AIDS are from 30 to 49. This could be attributed to the fact that the majority of Asian women start having sexual relations later than some other populations. The age difference also brings up the possibility that at least half the cases are probably first generation in this country or more recent immigrants. The cultural impact of immigration must be taken into consideration when approaching the issue of AIDS prevention among Asians and Pacific Islanders.

Another interesting statistic is that the transmission rate from blood transfusions is much higher than for other groups. Because of the incubation period, we can assume this could be from blood that has not been tested in Asia, as well as blood that wasn't tested here.

But also, these statistics may be affected by the level of denial that exists about AIDS. It's more acceptable to have become infected through a blood transfusion than through drugs or risky sexual behaviors. Also, some doctors in Asian communities are woefully ignorant about AIDS. Some doctors won't even treat or admit to treating people who are HIV positive. The doctor may have identified a case as a result of a transfusion. We can't be sure of the accuracy because of cultural attitudes.

There are more CDC-reported cases of AIDS among Asians and Pacific Islanders in the United States than in all the Asian countries and Pacific Islands that have reported cases to the World Health Organization. This can be attributed to the increased availability of testing here, but it also may be because of denial, or a yet to be proven scientific difference, or some other difference.

One of the major reasons for collecting statistics is to show how and among what peoples the disease has spread. In addition, the data collected serve as a teaching tool, to help people understand when they might be at highest risk when participating in certain behaviors.

Cultural Barriers to Preventing AIDS

The generation of immigration is crucial. No matter how long they've been here or when they arrived, first-generation persons usually stay in residential, cultural and language-based, close-knit societies with traditions of the country of origin; that is, no dating, or, in the extreme, arranged marriages. Homosexuality is not often discussed in many Asian cultures, but that is not true of all. Some countries openly recognize their homosexual men and lesbians. The reluctance, however, to speak of sex and drugs is even more difficult to overcome if cases of white or other ethnic group risk factors are openly portrayed in the media, and Asian cases are dismissed as "other" or as an asterisked footnote.

Particular issues affecting Asians must be addressed. These issues include, but are not limited to, reaffirming the efficacy of male-to-female transmission and the necessity for the protection of women of Asian ancestry who are the prey of visiting businessmen and the military, in their own countries as well as in the United States. Younger women and boys often engage in prostitution in order to contribute to the economic stability of the family, particularly those who have migrated to bigger cities and are without skills needed to survive in a higher-density urban area. In addition to prostitution for profit, companionship and marriage are very often intertwined, and the motivation is not always simply financial. The problem of the sex industry is that if the women are not aware of their risk factors, and the men are not about to use condoms, then they're in serious trouble.

Some of the statistics show that in particular areas where the sex industry has been flourishing, such as the Philippines and Thailand, the cases of HIV infection are high. Neither the World Health Organization nor the United States breaks these statistics down by gender, so it's hard to tell if the sex industry is involving more young men or young women. But it's still a problem where tourism is concerned.

In addition, in Asian and Pacific Islander cultures, childbearing is extremely important. Children are a way to continue a line of ancestry, respecting those who are the elders of the community. Since condoms interfere with childbearing, they are less likely to be accepted as a means to prevent HIV transmission. In the sex industry, young men are often just as preferred as young women. Attitudes about working in the sex industry, homosexuality, and childbearing are all very complex cultural issues, and do not engender simplistic responses. Therefore, the person teaching about HIV must be sensitive to and aware of cultural differences. It would be easy to dismiss the entire subcontinent of Asia and the Islands as homophobic, but that's too simplistic.

Over the last couple of years, the Asian cases of AIDS have doubled every 10 months. This makes education a critical issue. Dismissing the need for education because "the numbers are so low" flies in the face of how public health usually operates. After all, prevention is the only thing that can stop AIDS. New York City finally has come out with a little brochure that provides some resources. It's in English, but the cover is in five different languages. Another problem is that there aren't translators who have been provided with a sensitivity to AIDS and the subtleties of different cultures. Coming from cultures where stigmatization is feared, Asian people could be particularly drawn to the anonymity of a hotline. But New York state doesn't have a single person who can answer a question in any Asian or Pacific Island language. New York City has one person who speaks Chinese. This is a serious deficiency and is all the more critical because they don't have even have a full list of referrals. The highest number of HIV cases is Filipino, and there's nobody who speaks Tagalog or any other Philippine language hired by the City Board of Education or the City Department of Health to teach about HIV.

What We Need

The number of Asians and Pacific Islanders involved in AIDS work has grown. Two Asians attended the first Minority AIDS Conference in 1987, but in 1989 there were about 60. An Asian/Pacific Islander AIDS Coalition has been started in New York City. The first step is to learn who we are. We aren't all at the same level of ability to do AIDS education. The AIDS educator who has been hired for New York City is a man. There are a lot of women who simply will not talk to a man about these issues. It's totally insensitive not to have somebody who could respond to the needs of women.

There are excellent brochures developed by Asian/Pacific Islander organizations on the West Coast: for example, the Association of Asian/Pacific Community Health Organizations (AAPCHO), which has affiliates in San Francisco, Los Angeles, Hawaii, and Chinatown in New York. The federal government could use its brochures and pay to modify and distribute them to be appropriate in different communities. Why should everyone have to reinvent the wheel? Radio needs to be utilized, as it is a major form of communication. But education also needs to be one to one. People won't talk about AIDS in a group, and won't show up at a public meeting. Education has to be subsumed into the women's church group, sewing circle, or neighborhood women's auxiliary.

There's a whole denial of sex, let alone a denial of this disease. There's the problem of new immigrants wanting to fit into this country. They're not going to raise questions. Teenagers are particularly at risk because of peer pressure. Yet there's no information for them about dating, much less about safer sex.

The major task is first to educate public health officials who determine policy and then the people who implement the policy in lower-level education departments. This may mean providing an annotated abbreviated lesson in history, culture, geography, language, sexual customs, and sensitivity.

About the Author

Suki Ports founded the Minority AIDS Task Force in New York City in 1986. She is of third-generation Japanese descent.
Based on a discussion with Marion Banzhaf.

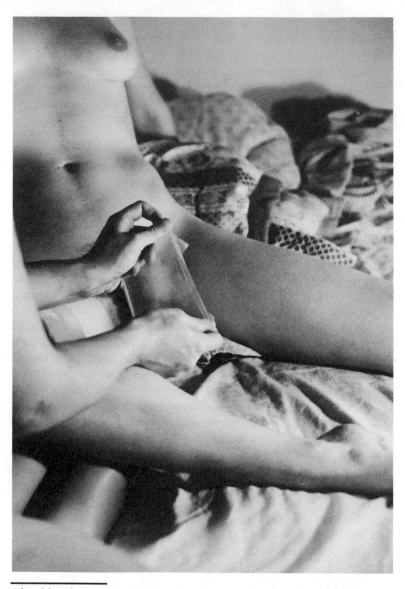

A dental dam about to be used. Photograph used in the development of the poster, "See Jane Put a Dental Dam on Sue."

Photo by Suzanne Wright

Lesbians in the AIDS Crisis

ZOE LEONARD

Lesbians have been absent from most discussion of HIV infection. The most common attitude seems to be that AIDS is not a lesbian problem. In the dominant media we are consistently portrayed as the "lowest-risk group," leading many people to believe that lesbians just don't get AIDS. Educational materials do not include information geared towards lesbians, nor do they ever discuss the possibility of woman-to-woman transmission. On the one hand, it is often implied that women who show concern or fear are alarmist. (One journalist went so far as to suggest that lesbians had AIDS envy.[1]) On the other hand, there seems to be a great deal of confusion among lesbians as to how we are at risk and what precautions we should take.

As lesbians we are affected by AIDS in many ways. There are lesbians who have AIDS. There have been several documented cases of women with HIV infection where the only possible route of transmission was sex with an HIV-positive woman. Lesbians are also subjected to the increased homophobia and bias-related violence occurring "in response" to the AIDS crisis. Some of us, who have gay male friends, have seen close friends die. Many lesbians are dedicated and outspoken AIDS activists and are building coalitions and working towards a feminist health movement and nationalized health care.

The Ways We Are at Risk

The idea that we are not at risk for HIV infection is not based on medical fact, but rather on a number of deep-rooted misconceptions about the way dykes live and how we have sex. For example, Dr. Charles Schable of the Centers for Disease Control (CDC) told *Visibilities,* a lesbian magazine, that it isn't neccessary to study lesbians because "lesbians don't have much sex."[2] The truth is that lesbians who engage in risky behavior are at risk for HIV infection. And there are lesbians who have AIDS.

Lesbians are not an isolated community: there are lesbians who shoot drugs and share needles, there are lesbians who have been married, who have babies, who are in prisons, who have sex for money, who get raped. When examining the AIDS epidemic, it becomes obvious that stereotypes are useless: it's not who you are that puts you at risk, it's what you do.

Many lesbians occasionally have sex with men, or have done so in the recent past. According to an ongoing Kinsey study, 46 percent of the self-identified lesbians surveyed reported having sex with a man since 1980.[3] There are women who were heterosexually identified and were having sex with men back in the early days of the epidemic, when it was widely believed that "straight people couldn't get it." There are also women who identify as straight, but occasionally have sex with other women, without perceiving the lesbian sex as a potential risk activity. Some lesbians have sex with gay or bisexual men and have reported very high-risk activities, such as unprotected anal intercourse.

Identifying as a lesbian will not change the realities of transmission through unsafe needle sharing. There are dykes who shoot drugs and share needles, and the lesbian community has to acknowledge that. Among female intravenous drug users (IVDUs), a fairly high percentage report having had sex with other women—as high as 19.6 percent according to the Urban Health study in San Fransisco.[4] In a related study, 26 out of 28 lesbian IVDUs had female partners who were also IVDUs; they could be at risk of contracting HIV through multiple means of transmission.[5]

Lesbians are at risk through alternative (artificial) insemination. At the IV International Conference on AIDS, Michael Rekart of Great Britain presented two confirmed cases of HIV transmission from an infected donor to the recipient of the sperm.[6] Dr. Ted Ellerbrock of the CDC cites four women in Australia who have contracted HIV in this way.[7]

Then there is the issue of woman-to-woman sexual transmission. According to Dr. Ellerbrock, female-to-female transmission is "biologically plausible,"[8] and there have been several documented cases. As early as 1984, a report was published about a lesbian who died of AIDS; both she and her partner denied needle use or sexual contact with men.[9] In 1986, another case was reported which involved an IV drug user and her lover. Both had AIDS, and all routes of transmission except sexual contact between the women had been ruled out. "Patient #2 reported having digital and oral contact with Patient #1's vagina and oral contact with her anus. Contact occurred during Patient #1's menses, and both women had vaginal bleeding as a result of traumatic sexual activities."[10] Another case involved a Filipina lesbian; it is presumed that she acquired HIV through performing cunnilingus.[11] A study conducted in New York with 31 infected lesbians found that 16 of them were IVDUs, 12 had had sex with infected men, and one had had a blood transfusion. Two of the women had no risk factor other than sex with other women.[12] In December 1989, doctors at Cornell reported another case of an HIV-positive lesbian. She has been in a monogamous relationship since 1980. Her lover is an ex-IVDU who has AIDS; her only sexual contact has been cunnilingus with her lover, and she has no personal history of drug use.[13]

In addition, there is a case of HIV being transmitted from a woman to a man through cunnilingus.[14] He says he never knowingly went down on her during her period. Although this case involves a heterosexual couple, the implications for lesbians are clear. Until evidence is presented to the contrary, unprotected oral sex between women cannot necessarily be considered safe.

Lack of Information and Research on Woman-to-Woman Transmission

Among the women with AIDS in the CDC's records, 100 report having had sex with other women.[15] However, for at least three reasons, this should not be taken as an accurate count. First, the CDC compiles its data from the reports of physicians across the country. It is very likely that most women will be assumed to be straight, and will never even be asked if they have had sex with other women. In fact, the case reporting forms are often filled out in the patient's absence. If you don't ask the questions, you won't get the answers. The case reporting forms are often illegible or incomplete. In fact, the CDC found it impossible to categorize nearly 700 out of 5,000 women because they couldn't determine their sexual behaviors from the report forms.[16] No one knows how many lesbians have AIDS, let alone how many are HIV infected.

Second, the CDC lists risks for exposure to HIV "hierarchically." In other words, if you are a lesbian IVDU with an IVDU partner, the possibility of woman-to-woman transmission would be ignored and you would be counted solely as an IVDU, even if you never shared needles. Men's "risk groups" now take into account multiple exposure risks. It is impossible to track women's risks accurately without reporting methods that are more inclusive and that acknowledge the possibility of multiple exposure.

A third factor complicating the collection of data on lesbians and AIDS is the very high chance of women being misdiagnosed. If you are considered to be in a "low-risk group" by your doctor, she or he may not consider HIV infection as a possibility.

We can only determine how efficient transmission of HIV between women is if data collection methods and medical studies are conducted more thoroughly and accurately. The doctors at the CDC seem satisfied that transmission between women is "not very efficient." Not only do we need more studies on lesbian sex practices, we need more information about HIV in menstrual blood, vaginal and cervical secretions, and other discharges. We also need to know more about the possible inhibitory qualities of saliva on HIV. Since transmission through oral sex and other sexual activities between women cannot be ruled out, all educational materials and safer-sex guidelines must include information pertinent to lesbians. We must learn from the history of the AIDS epidemic, and recognize the need for prevention in the lesbian community, rather than rely on flawed "low-risk group" analysis.

Assessing Our Risk

Sex between women is often thought of as soft core by its very nature, barely definable as sex at all. Yet lesbian sex routinely involves the exchange of body fluids and regularly serves to pass infections such as chlamydia, trichomonas, and gardnerella from one woman to another. HIV has been found in vaginal secretions and in menstrual blood, as well as in discharge from yeast infections. Many lesbians have oral-genital sex (cunnilingus). We may use our fingers, which might have small cuts or abrasions, we may share sex toys, or have sex that draws blood. One 1983 study comparing the sex habits of lesbians and straight women showed that the lesbians were far more sexually active.[17] Lesbians also spent 50 percent more time on oral activities (cunnilingus, rimming, kissing) than did the heterosexual women.[18] A 1979 study of 286 lesbians reported that one in four had experienced sadomasochism, and half preferred nonmonogamy.[19]

Because lesbians are repeatedly told that we are not at risk, very few dykes have adopted safe-sex techniques. In addition, our safe-sex needs are not being met. Although dental dams are a promising barrier method for oral sex, as are gloves for manual-genital contact, they have not been tested for effectiveness. Condom companies should make barriers from the same latex as condoms, which would be thinner and more sensitive than those now available. Dams should also be larger so that they are easier to hold in place.

Rather than panicking or seeking false reassurance, we need to learn to assess our risk more accurately, to examine our behaviors and the behaviors of our partners honestly. We are perhaps most at risk by denying our risk.

Dykes in the AIDS Community, Dykes in the AIDS Movement

Lesbians with HIV infection, like straight women, may have a hard time fitting into the "AIDS community." Many women feel awkward going to places where they are the only female clients. In fact, it is sometimes hard for women PWAs to find adequate medical care, especially gynecological care. Many of the support groups and services are provided basically for and by gay men, so female PWAs are often even more isolated than male PWAs.

As well as not fitting into the medical and social service system very well, lesbian PWAs also face painful and humiliating problems: family rejection (of either the PWA or her lover) and verbal or physical abuse from homophobic and AIDS-phobic individuals, on the street, at work, or even in the hospital.

Although we are understudied, and virtually invisible to the public eye, dykes have a long history of being politically active and have brought tremendous energy to the AIDS activist movement. There are some feminists, in fact, who feel that we have devoted too much energy to AIDS, that it is drawing energy away from "lesbian issues," and that we should disassociate ourselves from the crisis. But AIDS is a lesbian issue. By bringing our experiences to the AIDS activist movement, we broaden discussion. AIDS activism is not just about getting experimental drugs into PWAs' bodies, but it is also a movement for social change with a feminist agenda. We address health care as a whole, and recognize the need for responsible sex education, informed decision making, and nationalized health care.

Demands

- More accurate, inclusive case reporting.
- Multiple-risk categories for women.
- More research into lesbian sex.
- More research into women's body fluids.
- Better latex barriers produced by condom companies for women.

Acknowledgments

Thank you to Patricia Case, Donna Raskovage, and Denise Ribble.

Notes

1. Darrell Yates Rist, "The Deadly Costs of an Obsession," *The Nation*, February 13, 1989, p. 181.
2. Lee Chiaramonte, "Lesbian Safety and AIDS: The Very Last Fairy Tale," *Visibilities*, January-February 1988, p. 6.
3. Donna Minkowitz, "Safe and Sappho: An AIDS Primer for Lesbians," *Village Voice*, February 21, 1989, p. 21.
4. John Watters, Urban Health Study, personal communication, January 1990.
5. Patricia Case, Urban Health Study, Director of Lesbian AIDS Project, personal communications, December 1989-January 1990, regarding "The Social Context of AIDS Risk Behavior Among IV Drug Using Lesbians in San Fransisco," Patricia Case, Moher Downing, Bonnie Ferguson, et al., unpublished.
6. Michael L. Rekart, "HIV Transmission by Artificial Insemination," Abstract #4026, IV International Conference on AIDS, Stockholm, Sweden, June 12-16, 1988.
7. Ted Ellerbrock, M.D., Centers for Disease Control, personal communication, December 1989.
8. Ellerbrock, personal communication.
9. M. T. Sabatini, K. Patel, and R. Hirschman, "Kaposi's Sarcoma and T-Cell Lymphoma in an Immunodeficient Woman: A Case Report," *AIDS Research*, 1984, Vol. 1, pp. 135-137.
10. M. Marmor, L. R. Weiss, M. Lyden, et al., "Possible female to female transmission of human immunodeficiency virus" (letter), *Annals of Internal Medicine*, 1986, Vol. 105, p. 969.
11. O. T. Monzon and J. M. Capellan, "Female-to-female transmission of HIV," *Lancet*, 1987, Vol. 2, pp. 40-41.
12. Denise Ribble, Community Health Project, personal communication, December 1989, regarding "HIV Infection in Lesbians," Ribble, Marte, and Kelly, poster presentation at IV International AIDS Conference.
13. Samuel Perry, Lawrence Jacobsberg, and Karen Fogel, "Orogenital Transmission of Human Immunodeficiency Virus (HIV)," *Annals of Internal Medicine*, 1989, Vol. 111, no. 11, p. 951.
14. P. G. Spitzer, N. J. Weiner, "Transmission of HIV infection from a woman to a man by oral sex," *New England Journal of Medicine*, 1989, Vol. 320, p. 251.
15. Ellerbrock, personal communication.
16. Dr. Peter Drotman, Centers for Disease Control, personal communication, January 1990.
17. Chiaramonte, "Lesbian Safety and AIDS," p. 7.
18. Chiaramonte, "Lesbian Safety and AIDS."
19. Chiaramonte, "Lesbian Safety and AIDS."

Too Much Denial

CYNTHIA ACEVEDO

Just before I released the shutter, my lover suddenly asked would I make a panel for her if she died of AIDS. I felt a chill squeeze my heart, and I rushed my response back quickly, "Jesus, what kinda thing is that to say!" Never did I imagine that this moment would come back to haunt me as it has.

It was already late in the afternoon, and the bright glare of the sun was defiant before it began to set. Central Park was the site for the New York City Names Quilt panels. We had been hours late in arriving. Although I had tried getting my lover out of bed since morning, by mid-afternoon there had been little sign of her being ready. It was not until months later that the real reason for her incessant fatigue would become clear.

Four months later...it was the tail end of summer; I was sitting in the waiting room of the Corona public health station. My senses half dulled from the smell of disinfectant, and the other half completely terrorized by anxiety. It had been nearly a full hour that Moon had been away for her results. Moon and I had been together for nearly three years; she wanted more than anything to have a baby. It had been my idea that she have herself tested because IV drugs had been a part of her past. I had never doubted that Moon's results would be negative, so what was the delay? I remember us both racing out of the station onto the street when a fearless rain had driven everyone for cover. We stood there in the rain crying, completely lost for what to say or do next. I wanted to run and hide. I wanted to disappear, but there was no place to go and no one who could help us.

Before Moon's test I remember leaving ACT UP's Safer Sex Forum for Lesbians both annoyed and triumphant. What an absolute horror, I thought; could there really be something to all of this talk about lesbians and AIDS? The implications of what this meant were staggering. The idea that to eat pussy you now needed a baggy, Saran Wrap, or a barrier was more than I was willing to consent to, and certainly not in line with what these women wanted to hear. I remember the haunting analogy, "Let's not allow what happened in the gay male community to happen in our community." My relationships had been monogamous, and I had a pretty good idea of what my ex-lovers' past histories were like, or so I thought. Much of what the forum's facilitator said made perfect sense, from her risk assessment of sexual behaviors (a laundry list of common high-risk sexual behaviors), which everyone did miserably with, to the menu of new safer sexual practices to replace the high-risk behaviors. The objective of all this was to demonstrate that since the lesbian community was not a closed one, you had to also assume that neither was it free from risk.

Over the next months I had begun to experience tremendous anxiety over Moon's HIV status. Moon seemed completely defiant and determined that she would see to the state of her own affairs as she saw fit. Weeks turned into months and there was still no sign of her intentions concerning any type of treatment plan. She went on to deny her positive test results for almost a full year and became near reckless with her health. I knew that she was terrified; oftentimes she would stay up or wake up during the night, thinking that if she did this she could keep herself from having night sweats. There were now two worlds that emerged, and one clearly had little to do with the other. This virus living inside her was controlling everything; sometimes it seemed like there was an "us vs. them" thinking going on between us. After all, how much could I possibly understand anyway? It seemed as though the more Moon chose to ignore that she had tested positive, the more compelled I felt to encourage her to do something, anything at all.

When the heat between us became too great, she would attend her support group. But she was only going in order to defuse my threats, and so she was devoid of any conviction to be a part of the group. I remember feeling impotent and useless. No matter what I tried, I just could not get her to meet with me halfway on anything in terms of her health or our relationship together. My rage was becoming blinding. Whatever I tried was of little consequence. It seemed inconceivable to me for Moon to refuse my help. What was I doing wrong? The words enabler and codependent meant nothing at all to me; I could feel myself becoming sick with worry and terribly isolated. It was so difficult for us to share our fears with each other.

I remember naively thinking that if there were any saving grace to be had through all of this it was in discovering that Moon was positive before she was symptomatic. The issue of safer sex had reemerged, this time not as an abstract notion, but as a matter of reality. We had stopped having sex; discussions about what we should do or how we should handle it were strained. Moon suggested that I sleep with other women and not tell her about it. As a solution this was unacceptable; the best option available was to try safer sex. We had started discussions around the advantages and disadvantages with safer sex. We were both aware that measures needed to be taken. My own personal misgivings surrounding the sterilization of lesbian sex were no longer valid. There could no longer be any denying the necessity for it. We now needed to protect each other by taking precautions and practicing safer sex. We had discussed and agreed that we now had to use barriers during sex and that everything would be just fine. I should have had more common sense.

I decided to take the initiative and begin by setting the mood. I decided to follow the idea of safer sex panties and bought us each sexy French underwear. I removed the gussets and replaced them with chocolate dental dams I purchased from the Community Health Project. This turned out to be a mistake. Although I thought that we had realistically discussed the need for using some form of protection, for both our sakes, there was no ongoing dialogue. I too felt uncomfortable and clumsy about these changes; I was eager to restore some balance into our relationship. I really thought this would help. What resulted was a fiasco.

My baby's feelings of isolation and contamination had suddenly escalated from nightmare to reality. Apparently she had not given serious thought to the idea after all. Although she agreed with me over the necessity for us to start using safer sex, she had never really considered the matter. Upon arrival of the big moment, she unwrapped the box containing this strange-looking underwear. She held it out to me quizzically, awaiting an explanation. I stood there, mute for a moment, and then began to explain. We had been avoiding sex for months. This had after all been very serious business. Well, after the initial shock, there was nothing left to do except to try them on. There we were wearing our new state-of-the-art safety underwear. My baby began to cry. I felt totally mortified, I did not know what to say. I pulled her up close to me and assured her that everything would work out, we just needed time and practice, and then we both cried.

Problems began to emerge; dental dams were never intended for oral sex. I could not achieve orgasm due to the density of the rubber. This really began to piss me off. We began using condoms instead of the dams. Although an improvement, they proved to be impractical and clumsy. There were many moments when I thought how much easier everything would be to just forget the barriers, even if only occasionally. Whenever I brought up the issue to Moon, she would have no part of it. We started having sex less and less frequently. Moon had stopped sleeping with me altogether. When she could no longer avoid giving me an explanation, she told me she felt like a germ and that it was better if we slept apart. This proved to be the source of some of our worst arguments.

Whenever the issue of safer sex came up, I would immediately begin to defend it, along with the necessity for all women to learn about it and to practice it. In place of my own conviction there was a void that kept me from facing the failure of this idea within my own relationship. It seemed to me that the strongest advocates of this idea were often the ones who didn't need to own their commitment fully.

My denial is similar to that of other lesbians. As our community has historically smoothed over the issues of substance abuse and bisexuality, we as lovers, caregivers, and friends must examine more closely and deliberately when and how we must practice safer sex. Each of us has our own process and set of priorities that must be identified and dealt with. It is truly a courageous thing to uncloud one's vision and not be afraid to alter one's ideals and behaviors when necessary.

Intravenous Drug Use, Women, and HIV

CATHERINE SAALFIELD

with CYNTHIA CHRIS, RACHEL LURIE, and MONICA PEARL

Intravenous drug use puts women at risk for HIV infection in a number of ways. The immediate risk from sharing IV needles is compounded by the risk of unprotected sex with IV drug users. Drug addiction demands attention that may preclude concern with HIV; people who shoot up may not have the money, time, energy, or desire to pay attention to good nutrition, bleaching needles, or preventing transmission of HIV. Intravenous drug users (IVDUs) experience an especially alienated relationship to the AIDS crisis and to the interventions that AIDS activists and service workers have provided.

Being drunk or stoned can inhibit our ability to be concerned with and to negotiate safer sex. For this reason, substance use can be considered a cofactor in the transmission of HIV. As well, alcohol, marijuana, heroin, cocaine and its derivatives (e.g., crack), amphetamines, barbiturates, synthetic drugs ("designer drugs": Ecstasy, crank, ice), and poppers (amyl or butyl nitrite) are immunosuppressive. Therefore, they may be considered cofactors in the development of HIV disease and may pose additional health risks for those already infected.

Heroin, speed, and cocaine can all be injected intravenously. Seroprevalence of HIV among those who shoot cocaine is much greater than those who shoot heroin, due, most likely, to the fact that intravenous cocaine users inject themselves as often as 30 to 40 times a day and will more frequently "boot" (pump the drug in and out between the vein and syringe, which increases blood-to-blood contact).

According to current statistics, IVDUs comprise 21 percent of all diagnosed people with AIDS in the United States. Approximately half of all women with AIDS are IVDUs. Approximately a third have been sexual partners of HIV-infected men who are thought to be IVDUs;

another 8 percent acquired HIV through an unknown transmission route. Such a large percentage of women whose risk factors are unknown indicates strongly that disregard for multiple modes of transmission makes it impossible to track women's exposure risk accurately.

Trying to untangle modes of transmission as they relate to women and intravenous drugs is difficult because a woman could be shooting unsafely and having unsafe sex with someone who is shooting unsafely, or she could only be having unsafe sex with someone who is shooting unsafely, or she could only be shooting up unsafely. The Centers for Disease Control (CDC) always seem to choose the most stigmatized transmission mode possible when categorizing AIDS cases. This is a general methodological problem in AIDS epidemiology and in mainstream AIDS discourse. Further, the CDC keeps statistics on multiple modes of transmission only for men; women are categorized exclusively by the mode of transmission thought to be most likely. Insofar as repeated exposure accelerates HIV replication, women must be educated about all the behaviors that put them at risk, not just the behaviors that are deemed more risky by arbitrary and skewed statistics.

Transmission Issues and Realities for Women Drug Users

There are additional cofactors in HIV transmission particular to drug use, other than unsafe needle use. For example, crack use can be considered a cofactor, in that many women with drug habits will perform sex for money or drugs and often will agree not to use a condom to get more money. Being high can significantly distort the importance of practicing safe sex.

Many IVDUs have had blood transfusions when hospitalized for problems that may be related to drug use, such as severe chronic anemia resulting from poor nutrition, violent injuries, or complications during childbirth that could cause hemorrhages. Until HIV testing of donated blood became routine in 1985, multiple transfusions presented some risk of HIV infection. Other immunosuppressive health conditions are also common in IVDUs, such as hepatitis B, which may put one at greater risk for HIV and which is also transmitted by sex or by intravenous injection.

IV Drug Use and HIV: What Is (Not) Known and What Is (Not) Being Done

Scapegoated as vectors of transmission, IVDUs are receiving attention only insofar as non-IV drug using populations are threatened. There is little consideration for their rights to health care and information. According to Edith Campbell of the Montefiore Methadone Maintenance Program, "IVDUs are a population that until now has not even been acknowledged as existing in terms of being entitled to any attention from the rest of society. Suddenly, because there's a threat coming through AIDS; everyone wants to know what's going on."[1]

Seroprevalence among IVDUs in New York City may be as high as 80 percent. In other cities, seroprevalence is as low as 4 percent (in Los Angeles) to 10 percent (in Atlanta).[2] These rates may be affected by the availability of substance abuse treatment, by whether or not over-the-counter sale of needles is legal, by access to needle exchange programs, and by the kinds of drugs and drug-using practices common in each community. Further study is necessary for activists and service providers to know which strategies are the most effective in slowing the rates of HIV transmission via IV drug use and thus, which to support.

Drug treatment programs may not have adequate services for people with AIDS, and AIDS service organizations often lack services and programs directed to IVDUs. There are so few drug treatment slots that those who want to quit drugs are often on waiting lists for months before they can begin treatment. But experimental drug trials for people with HIV frequently exclude active IVDUs and require former IVDUs to have been clean for long periods of time. Often researchers excuse this based on stereotypes of drug users, such as inability to keep appointments and poor personal hygiene and health.

According to Yolanda Serrano of the Association for Drug Abuse Prevention and Treatment (ADAPT), "Many substance abusers have been denied access to drug trials and have to claim to be gay or bisexual to get into a trial."[3] An IVDU who is HIV positive must have access to treatment for her or his HIV infection as well as her or his addiction.

While over half of the drug-using population in the United States is comprised of women, women constitute only 32 percent of those enrolled in treatment programs. Only about half of the 7,000 treatment programs nationwide provide female patients with child and obstetric care. Fewer than six drug treatment programs in the United States exist specifically for pregnant drug users and are essentially the only programs that will accept pregnant substance users at all. In many states, if treatment programs are full, a woman can be sent to a correctional facility even though she has committed no crime. Once there, she may not attend substance-abuse programs because she is not part of the official prison population.[4]

Treatment on Demand

The most effective strategy to slow the transmission of HIV would be immediate treatment on demand for chemical addiction. Such programs would have to include residential detoxification and counseling; methadone maintenance; chemical-free, alternative detox programs, such as acupuncture; and self-help groups, such as Narcotics Anonymous. Residential programs are the most expensive, but also are considered the most effective.

Guaranteed access to any of these programs includes transportation, help in filling out housing applications and welfare paperwork, day care for women with children, interpreters for people who don't speak English, and culturally sensitive education and counseling. Undocumented people must be given assistance and waivers for fees to acquire birth certificates and other identification that may be necessary for entering drug treatment programs. Finally, programs must eradicate the requirement for an address that homeless people may not be able to produce.

Needle Exchange Programs

Successful, government-backed needle exchange programs have been tried in the Netherlands, England, and the United States, notably in Tacoma, Washington, and Portland, Oregon. In 1988, a Needle Exchange and Education Program (NEEP) was begun in New York City; it was dismantled early in 1990. The bureaucracy that one had to wade through in order to participate severely limited its effectiveness; only about 300 people participated. IVDUs had to register by name, travel to the downtown exchange site that was across the street from a police station, give blood, and agree to drug treatment.

The notion of needle exchange is very controversial, but barring unlimited drug treatment programs, needle exchange remains a necessary battleground. It has been attacked by some of New York City's Black and religious leaders as encouraging drug use and thus representing genocide to affected communities. To counter this point of view, Yolanda Serrano says, "It's not the needle that gets people to use drugs; it's the high." ADAPT viewed the success of the NEEP in terms of how many IVDUs could get into treatment quickly. In fact, affirms Serrano, "One guy who joined the program got into drug treatment before he even needed to exchange a needle."[5]

Other needle exchange programs employ a more user-friendly approach, believing that to be at all effective, they must be street based, anonymous, and nonjudgmental. These unsanctioned programs exist in several cities. The people instigating exchanges generally see their work as a form of direct action and view the risks, such as arrest, as a part of saving lives.

Patricia Case, an activist and health care worker with Prevention Point Needle Exchange, an entirely volunteer group in San Francisco, explained that the project "started as a civil disobedience action" in 1988 by a group of health care workers, AIDS activists, and others. On their first night on the street, they exchanged three needles; now they exchange 2,500 a night. The program is an *exchange;* that is, people have to have a needle in order to get a new, clean one. While bleach is important, it is "an emergency measure" to be used when an IVDU doesn't have clean works. Case added that substance users are receptive to the exchange program: "They are interested in preventing HIV."

For Case and others involved in street-based needle exchange projects, the whole point is to save lives directly. "I started doing this so that I could sleep at night 20 years from now," she said, explaining that she had had a job giving HIV-antibody tests, and "couldn't give out one more positive test result without starting to give out needles." She noted that the seroprevalence rate among IVDUs in San Francisco is between 15 and 20 percent. "We couldn't wait to be like New York, where the seropositive rate is [at least] 65 percent, before doing something."[6]

Virtually every street-based needle exchange program has a comprehensive agenda that includes access to drug treatment on demand, outreach, and education. Prevention Point Needle Exchange's operation is based on the following goals: (1) to fight for drug treatment on demand; (2) to provide culturally and linguistically appropriate AIDS information and education; (3) to provide access to condoms, bleach, alcohol swabs, and other means of preventing HIV transmission; and (4) anonymous needle exchange.

Education

City and state authorities are merely treating the symptom when they launch their tired and inappropriate campaigns to counter the spread of HIV among IVDUs. What we need are thorough, accurate, and culturally sensitive educational campaigns about safer sex and cleaning needles. "Culturally sensitive" materials must emerge from the targeted community, and must recognize cultural values, such as gender roles and familial structure, as they relate to sexuality and drug use. According to the executive director of the community-based organization Loisaida and former executive director of the Hispanic

A certain kind of brochure will reach one kind of person. A certain kind of brochure in a certain language will reach yet another person. And then there are brochures that will reach no one because they either can't read or don't read...Even though there's a lot of lip service paid to the diversity, there's no real recognition of it and no communication system in place because that would require political recognition of these groups.[7]

A recent study of 263 men and 126 women who were arrested in Santa Clara County, California, from August to September 1989, showed that while only 19 percent of the men continued to share needles after receiving information about HIV transmission, 42 percent of the women continued to share.[8] Perhaps women face greater difficulty in acquiring new works; perhaps we face greater difficulty convincing those with whom we share to change their practices, due to economic dependence and other factors. One has to ask if the information reaching the women is relevant to their lives and drug-using practices.

Demands

The New York City Department of Health threatened to stop funding ADAPT in May 1990 if they continued to provide even just bleach to their clients. We demand unconditional funding for local drug treatment and advocacy programs, especially those run by recovering addicts, such as ADAPT and Promesa, Inc. They need money to provide counseling for substance users of all types, medical referrals for people with HIV infection, and other relevant and invaluable support services. Because they are already established and trusted in the target communities, these organizations are best suited to take on such tasks.

As AIDS activists and people with AIDS, we need more accurate and explicit information about drug use and about sex. We must make expanded treatment and support services for IVDUs an integral part of our activist agenda. We also need to step back and ask why substance users are perceived and treated as criminals; why poor people and people of color are the majority of IVDUs in this society; why people in prisons are primarily people of color and poor people, many of whom are substance users; and who exactly is profiting from the drug epidemic.

Is there some political dividend or benefit in the fact that thousands upon thousands if not millions of ghetto youths who are potential political activists who have everything to gain by radical change in this country are taken out of the political scene when they go on crack or cocaine or heroin?[9]

Notes

1. Jean Carlomusto and Alexandra Juhasz, *Living with AIDS: Women and AIDS*, videotape (New York: Gay Men's Health Crisis, 1988).
2. John A. Newmeyer, Ph.D., "The Epidemiology of HIV Among Intravenous Drug Users," in *Face to Face: A Guide to AIDS Counseling*, James W. Dilley, Cheri Pies, Michael Helquist, eds. (San Francisco: AIDS Health Project, University of California San Francisco, 1989), p. 109.
3. Chris Bull, "AIDS Doc Blasts City on Treatment Access," *Outweek*, September 24, 1989, no. 14, p. 17.
4. Susan Diesenhouse, "Drug Treatment is Scarcer than Ever for Women," *The New York Times*, January 7, 1990, p. 26.
5. Yolanda Serrano, personal communication.
6. Patricia Case, personal communication, January 1990.
7. Carlomusto and Juhasz, *Living with AIDS*.
8. Anthony Villalobos, "Women Twice as Likely to Continue Sharing Needles," *Gay Community News*, November 26-December 2, 1989, p. 2.
9. Philip Agee, "Anticommunism in the U.S.: History and Consequences," lecture delivered at conference, Harvard University (November 1988). Audiotape available from Institute for Media Analysis.

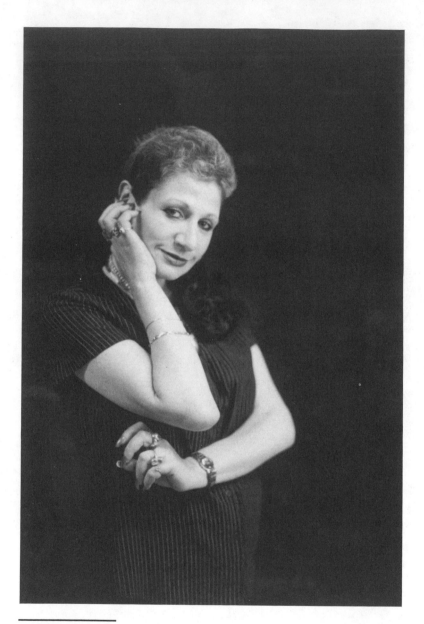

Iris de la Cruz
Photo by Zoe Leonard

An Excerpt from
"Sex, Drugs, Rock-n-Roll, and AIDS"[1]

IRIS DE LA CRUZ

I remember seeing the prostitutes on Third Avenue. I started getting high with them and before long I was out there turning tricks. I thought it was great. I had enough money to take care of both my heroin habit and my child and to maintain an apartment on East 14th Street. I walked to work at night! By this time I was taking courses at the School of Visual Arts and shooting up before school in the bathroom. My daughter was attending day care (which was affiliated with the Puerto Rican Socialist Party—old habits die hard). And I thought I was doing all right.

When I started hustling, most of the women were white. Nobody turned a trick for less than $25, and if you were picked up for loitering, they let you out in the morning. They even had a squad of cops, known as the "pussy posse," to round up the whores. I thought I had it made. I liked the feeling of power having men honk their horns as I walked the streets. And the idea that these men thought I was pretty enough to pay me for sex was a big ego boost. This went on for years with the drug habit increasing subtly.

During this time I started writing and got a job writing columns on drugs and sex for men's magazines. This was the mid-1970s, and drugs and disco were considered very chic. All the good parties had lines of coke on coffee tables, and sex clubs were making millions. The party continued. Same faces, different drugs. My drug usage escalated. I dropped out of college and sent my daughter to San Francisco to live with her father. I still kept writing.

My editor set up a meeting with a woman who was organizing prostitutes out on the West Coast, and she asked me if I was interested in reviving P.O.N.Y. (Prostitutes of New York). My best friend had just been found nude, under the Brooklyn Bridge, with her throat cut. We used to watch each other's backs out on the stroll. Hookers needed to be protected, since it was obvious the police and government thought we were expendable. I became the spokesperson for P.O.N.Y. and did all kinds of interviews. The media has always been enthralled with articulate "street people." I kept the ratings up. This went on for about a year while I spent more and more time in shooting galleries. Finally, the unions started getting interested in prostitutes, and P.O.N.Y. started becoming enmeshed in politics. I walked away.

A couple of years passed, and my drug habit became the only thing I was interested in. I lost my apartment and was basically living in shooting galleries. I was still hustling, but the wait between tricks became longer and longer. I looked and acted like your basic run-of-the-mill junkie. I had amassed 26 arrests, two of them for second-degree assault. I had meant it when I said that no one was ever gonna beat me. I became real good with a knife and felt nothing cutting someone. I felt nothing anyway. If I called my daughter and any feelings of love or regret came up, I would sedate myself. My life consisted of getting high (I was now addicted to heroin, methadone, sleeping pills, and tranquilizers) and turning tricks. Emotions were not something I wanted to deal with. I used to pray to die. I'd overdose almost every month and then raise hell with hospital staff for reviving me. I tried getting into drug treatments, but they were overcrowded and had waiting lists.

This was a very exciting time in my life. Too bad I wasn't there to experience it. I had a boyfriend I really did love (I just wasn't wild about myself). So there was someone to watch my back and get high with. But I was getting tired. There is nothing more pitiful than an old junkie whore.

It was about this time that I started noticing that a lot of my friends were getting sick and dying. When I had to be hospitalized for pelvic inflammatory disease, the rage kicked up again. I returned to the streets with a vengeance and became known as La Blanca Loca (the crazy white woman). I fought with everyone until in a spaced-out rage I stabbed a man that tried to rip me off.

I was given one and one-half to three years. I kicked all the drugs in jail, complete with convulsions, vomiting, and diarrhea. I hated being locked up, and it occurred to me that the main reason people are locked away is because they're a threat either to themselves or to society. On drugs, I was both. I copped to a program after spending eight months dealing with the insanity the New York State Department of Corrections is notorious for. It was time to start over.

I stayed in treatment for about nine months and learned some very important things, like how to channel my rage, and loving support, and encounter groups. I learned how to accept and give love. I also learned why so many of my friends were dying. We started losing people in the program. The enemy finally had a name. It was AIDS.

After I left treatment I took a course and got my license as an emergency medical technician. I had been drug free for some time and was making Narcotics Anonymous meetings. So I worked as an EMT with plans to someday go through medical school. After years of destructive behavior, I really felt I had to pay back for the very fact that I was still alive. I guess it's true what they say about the Lord protecting fools and children. So I worked, and tried to ignore the little things that kept cropping up, such as the white stuff in my mouth and the fatigue.

I used to transport AIDS patients a lot, since I was the only one that didn't give the dispatcher a hard time about it. By this time they were finding out that the disease wasn't airborne, and it was only transmitted by bodily fluids. So I would wear gloves but refused to wear a mask or "suit up" to transport AIDS patients. Emergency Room nurses would run all kinds of guilt trips about what I was bringing home to my family. I once had a big fight with a charge nurse after I suctioned a patient in the E.R. with PCP. He was left for over an hour all congested. Medical staff, on the whole, resented AIDS patients. The feeling was that they were all faggots and dope fiends and deserved what they got. By this time, I knew what the signs and symptoms were. I knew I was positive for the AIDS virus.

I was still working, even though I was tired all the time. Finally I had a patient go into cardiac arrest in the back of an ambulance. The man had a urinary obstruction and was semicomatose. I panicked and started CPR without a mask. I found out later he had active tuberculosis. A few weeks later, after working with soaring fevers, I had to be hospitalized.

My temperature was spiking up to 105.5 degrees, and the nurses were telling my mother to stay with me because I would not make it through the night. I was delirious and spoke with my father and grandmother. They're both dead. But I made it; I guess I'm too much of a bitch to die.

I got out of the hospital 90 days later looking like the national AIDS poster child. I spent the next ten months getting my weight and strength back. Locked in my mom's house, I felt like a germ. Back to feeling ugly and unloved. I didn't want to be touched because I felt unclean. In this society women's bodies are unclean and have to be deodorized before they're acceptable. So now, on top of everything,

I was diseased. My mother wouldn't hear it. She kept hugging me despite the fact that I shied away, began attending a mothers' group, and forced me to go out. My first time on a train I sat there looking at lovers and families and thinking that these options are closed to me. I would look at the person next to me and think, "Would they still sit next to me if they knew I had AIDS?"

I started attending a group for women with HIV. I felt like I was the only woman in the world with AIDS. It was all gay white men. This group changed that.

All of a sudden I discovered other women with the virus. There were Black women, white women, Latinas, rich women, and poor women. There were addicts and transfusion women. They were mothers and sisters and lovers and daughters and grandmothers. Some were militant lesbians and others were Republicans (imagine that! Even Republicans get AIDS). And we were all connected by the virus. Outside differences became trivial; feelings and survival were everyone's main concern. And I learned that there was still a lot of love left in me. The rage mellowed.

I was diagnosed with AIDS two years ago. I kept attending the women's group until the leader left. Then I took over the facilitator's role along with my best friend, Helen, who has ARC. A few months ago I started a group for bi- and heterosexuals dealing with HIV. I do AIDS outreach and education. I teach safer sex and show addicts how to clean their works. I encourage them to seek treatment. The rage that burned is now a hot anger. I've been to too many funerals with this disease. I'm tired of the newly diagnosed being made to feel dirty. I'm tired of my people being neglected and left dying on the streets. My child is now 19 and we're very close. The legacy I want to leave her is for her to remember her mama was a survivor. She survived drugs and she survived her own worst enemy, which was herself. And she taught others survival. She may or may not have survived AIDS, but she kicked ass while she was here.

Notes

1. This article is excerpted from a longer, unpublished essay.

Teenagers

RACHEL LURIE

Teenagers in the United States have long been besieged by the contradictions of a society that gives them very little credit. On the verge of adulthood, teenagers are not allowed information that will shape the types of adults they could become. Instead, adult society restricts the information given to teens and then punishes them for making the wrong choices, never thinking that the answer is to give teenagers more information in the first place.

Nowhere is this contradiction more evident than in the area of teenage sexuality. Once again, teenagers fall victim to the denial and self-righteousness of an adult mainstream which itself has severe problems talking honestly and realistically about sex and sexuality. The forces that control information, from education in the schools to public service messages on TV or on buses and subways, are unwilling to start from the premise that teenagers desire sex, teenagers have sex, and teenagers, like all of us, are at risk for HIV. Drugs are given similar treatment and talked about only in vague and moralistic terms. But young people do use them. Teenagers are more likely to have sex and use drugs than to have access to adequate information about either.

In October 1989, reports came out that highlighted the concern of those who had been doing AIDS education work with teenagers for the past several years. Shaken awake by a 40 percent increase in adolescent AIDS cases in the last two years, health care professionals are now warning that the high level of HIV infection among teenagers "is going to be the next crisis" and that "it's going to be devastating."[1] Because HIV generally has a latency period of five to eight years or more between exposure and developing symptoms of HIV-related illness, the people who will be getting sick several years from now are those exposed today—many of them teens.

Also, in New York City, the male-to-female ratio of AIDS cases among adults is eight to one; with teenagers it is anywhere from three to one to virtually equal.[2] New York City statistics will be replicated throughout the United States if preventative measures are not taken.

Lack of information is a significant problem in leaving young people at risk for HIV infection. For young women, the powerlessness is felt in several other ways.

- Young women have been infected as a result of sexual abuse by HIV-positive men.
- Young female prostitutes are at risk because they are unable to demand condom use by their male customers.
- Young women are expected by their peers to be both hetero-sexual and sexually active. Many lesbian teenagers will have unprotected sex with a man in an effort to become pregnant and prove their femininity. Teenagers are not given the tools to demand that their partners use a condom every time.

About 70 percent of U.S. citizens have had sex before turning 18-years-old. One in ten teenagers contracts a sexually transmitted disease each year. One in ten teenage girls becomes pregnant.[3] It is more than clear that the prevailing "education" strategy of telling kids to "just say no," chiding them with a wink, and telling them to take a cold shower, is foolish at best, murderous at worst.

We know that more than 20 percent of those who have died of AIDS have been in their twenties, and with an incubation period of five to eight years or more, most of those were infected in their teenage years. Yet young people do not perceive themselves as being at risk for HIV infection, a major obstacle in any prevention strategy.

So who is working to educate teenagers about safer sex and risk assessment? Not the schools. There are a million students enrolled in the New York City public schools: one-eighth of the city's population. But when the Board of Education offers anything at all, it is too watered down to accomplish anything. The statewide Board of Regents has this frightening policy: "The Board of Regents views the use of condoms as *extremely high-risk behavior* (italics mine). The view that condoms should or can be used as a way to reduce the risk of transmission of AIDS should not be supported."[4]

Gerri Abelson, the director of New York City's AIDS education program in the public schools, argues that the best risk reduction is "delaying the onset of sexual activity" and is opposed to endorsing condom use because "if we do that, we have to teach kids how to use them."[5]

Nationwide, it's not much better. In a review of 18 curricula from school boards around the country, the Centers for Disease Control found that one quarter of them "did not address abstinence or condom use."[6]

Not surprisingly, studies on youth's awareness around HIV transmission and AIDS show ignorance, but not as much as the Board of Education would like. Kids do seek out information, and then share it with each other. When a group of ACT UP members distributed safe-sex literature, condoms, and dental dams outside of several New York high schools and middle schools in the spring of 1989, the kids came in droves, taking away thousands of pieces of literature and latex. Some school officials were as impressed as the ACT UP folks were and proposed formal presentations in the future, though one principal called the cops and another stood at the school's entrance with a garbage can to collect the condoms.[7]

When kids do get hold of contraceptives, they often don't use condoms. According to the Center for Population Options, "Only one-third of sexually active teens use contraception regularly, and less than one quarter of those who use contraception use condoms."[8] In a 1985 San Francisco survey, 40 percent of those queried did not know that using condoms lowers the risk of infection with the virus.[9]

Education in the schools is a major issue for activists to address. But many of the kids most at risk aren't in school anyway. Kids who survive on the street have often run away or been thrown out of homes where they were neglected or abused. They have risk factors that aren't connected only to drug use and sexual behavior but also to a social system that leaves them powerless. These kids, the most disenfranchised, have the highest rate of HIV infection. But often they're worried about their next meal, not a virus that may make them sick in eight or ten years.

There are also kids who live on the streets only on weekends and return home during the week, where they return to their regular partners and often won't use condoms.

The disempowerment that comes from being a teenager in an adult world is magnified by being a young woman in a sexist world. While women in general have so little access to treatment, teenagers have the additional strike against them of being minors. Young women need one-on-one and group counseling with peers that teaches them how to negotiate safer sex. Counselors also must recognize that teenagers don't always have choices. A high percentage of women and girls who are raped are teenagers. Any counseling program needs to look realistically at the lives of teenagers, what they do, what they want to do, and what they cannot control.

One thing is sure: kids want information, not browbeating. Moralizing won't save lives. Whether through school curricula, street outreach, or peer counseling, young people want real answers to real questions, information that allows them the dignity to make their own decisions.

Acknowledgments

This essay is based on one by Ann Northrop, appearing in the original ACT UP/NY Women and AIDS handbook.

Notes

1. Gina Kolata, "New Trends Alarming to Experts," *The New York Times,* October 8, 1989, p. 1.
2. Kolata, "New Trends," p. 1.
3. Center for Population Options, "AIDS and Adolescents: The Time for Prevention is Now" (October 1988), CPO, 1012 14th St. NW, Suite 1200, Washington, D.C. 20005.
4. Sandor Katz, "NY AIDS Education: Anti-Sex Fear Mongering," *Outweek,* July 3, 1989, p. 28.
5. Hetrick-Martin Institute literature, received from Ann Northrop.
6. Center for Population Options, "AIDS and Adolescents," p. 6.
7. Katz, "NY AIDS Education," p. 28.
8. Center for Population Options, "AIDS and Adolescents," p. 1.
9. Center for Population Options, "AIDS and Adolescents," p. 2.

Prison Issues and HIV: Introduction

KIM CHRISTENSEN

Most written material on the subject of HIV disease in prisons focuses on male prisoners; little statistical evidence has been gathered on incarcerated women. Two things, however, are clear. First, AIDS is growing rapidly as a cause of death in the prison system nationwide. As of June 1989, there were 36,855 women in federal and state prisons,[1] approximately 30,000 women in local jails,[2] and approximately another 600,000 on parole or probation.[3] Among prisoners in New York City and New York state, AIDS is now the leading cause of death.[4]

Second, a significant percentage of incarcerated women are known to be HIV positive. The New York State Commission on Corrections estimates that 17.4 percent of women entering prison in New York state are HIV positive. In addition, a large percentage of women prisoners have histories of IV drug use, a significant source of HIV transmission for women. In New York state, between 60 and 70 percent of entering prisoners are estimated to have IV drug-use histories.[5]

In New York state, incarcerated women diagnosed with AIDS live approximately half as long as their male counterparts.[6] The average survival time for women from AIDS diagnosis to time of death is between five and six months.[7] Given the lack of proper medical treatment in prison, entering prison is a virtual death sentence for many women PWAs with felony convictions.

Due to their relative isolation from public view, prisoners have often been subjected to procedures that violate their basic legal and human rights. This is especially true in the AIDS crisis, where mandatory HIV testing, segregation (quarantine), and other measures are routine in many prisons.

Surveys show that segregation (by result of HIV-antibody test) is common: according to a recent study, 41 percent of city and county jails segregate all seropositive inmates, and an additional 30 percent make case-by-case determinations. The incidence of segregation of prisoners with AIDS or ARC is still higher.[8]

Although such segregation is useless for stopping the spread of AIDS, "...segregation can be devastating for those prisoners subjected to it."[9] Keeping HIV-positive and other noncontagious prisoners out of the general prison population is "...punitive...with denial of access to the law library, jobs, education, recreation, visitation, the canteen, etc."[10] More importantly, nonparticipation in programming "...can prevent inmates from earning good time credit towards release."[11]

Alabama HIV-positive prisoners lost a federal class action suit when challenging the state's policy allowing mandatory testing of all prisoners without their knowledge or consent. Both female and male HIV-positive prisoners were quarantined and told that they had AIDS and were going to die. The judge ruled that quarantine was not a violation of the prisoners' First Amendment rights. Even the lack of medical attention was not redressed, and the judge went so far as to say that if Alabama provided quality medical care to prisoners, people with AIDS might break laws in order to receive "free" medical care in prison.[12] This case will be appealed, but the prisoners in isolation and without medical care in Alabama will probably not survive to see the outcome.

Currently, there are still no experimental drug trials in women's prisons, and AZT is considered "standard of care" treatment. Given the lack of effective, approved treatments for AIDS, experimental drug trials provide the only hope for many PWAs to prolong and improve the quality of their lives. For this reason, women PWAs in prison must have access to experimental drug trials, as well as compassionate use and investigational new drug (IND) protocols if they so choose.

At the same time that we advocate for prisoner access to experimental drugs, we must be aware that incarcerated people have been abused in experimental drug trials and "scientific" experiments in the past. (The Tuskegee Institute syphilis study on Black men is probably the most well known.) Since such studies can easily be hidden from public view, they must be carefully monitored by prisoner advocates.

Demands for Improving the Treatment of Imprisoned Women with AIDS

New legislation, class action suits, and other activities may be helpful in gaining PWA prisoners their rights. It is also essential to remember that outside pressure is almost always needed to change conditions inside the prison. The following demands must be made on city, state, and federal prison systems:

- Anonymous HIV-antibody testing for prisoners.
- Access to condoms and dental dams to prevent sexual transmission of HIV, and bleach to prevent unsafe needle use.
- Peer AIDS education and counseling to prevent violence against HIV-positive prisoners.
- Culturally sensitive AIDS education and counseling, in appropriate languages, and at various literacy levels, for the families of prisoners.
- AIDS education for correctional officers, prison administrators, and medical personnel.
- Confidential, state-of-the-art health care, including experimental drugs and prophylactic treatments, but prisoners must not be subjected to experimental treatments without their informed consent.
- Comprehensive health care support services for PWAs released on parole.
- Government appropriations for prisons to meet these demands.

One hopeful exception to the generally dismal state of prison AIDS care is the ACE (AIDS Counseling and Education) program at Bedford Hills Correctional Facility, a maximum security women's prison north of New York City. ACE was founded after a woman PWA was isolated in the infirmary and not allowed to join the general population. Several prisoners visited the PWA on a regular basis, and eventually decided to try to educate themselves and the rest of the prison population about AIDS. Peer counseling was disdained by many prison authorities on the grounds that only "experts" can talk about AIDS. But the prisoners persisted, and over the course of four years put together a curriculum that addresses, among other topics, HIV transmission, risk reduction, HIV testing, strategies for treatment, and social issues pertaining to women and AIDS. The selection that follows, written by the women of ACE, describes their struggle to create meaningful and effective AIDS peer education in a prison setting. The peer education approach, which stresses empowerment and building community, must be adopted by prisons across the country if their AIDS education programs are to be successful.

Acknowledgments

Deb Levine contributed to this essay.

Notes

1. Bureau of Justice Statistics, telephone inquiry, January 18, 1990.
2. Steven Whitman, Center for Urban Affairs, Northwestern University, personal communication, January 18, 1990.
3. Bureau of Justice Statistics, telephone inquiry, January 18, 1990.
4. Cathy Potler, "AIDS in Prison: A Crisis in New York State Corrections," New York State Commission of Corrections (1988), p. 6.
5. Potler, "AIDS in Prison," p. 13.
6. Potler, "AIDS in Prison," p. 13.
7. Barbara Santee, Ph.D., Women and AIDS Resource Network, "Women and AIDS: The Silent Epidemic" (June 1988).
8. Paul Albert, "AIDS in Jails and Prisons: What We Can Do," *The Exchange*, National Lawyers' Guild AIDS Network (1986), p. 1.
9. Alvin Bronstein, Executive Director of the National Prison Project of the ACLU, Testimony before the Subcommittee on Courts, Civil Liberties and the Administration of Justice Concerning Oversight Related to AIDS and the Criminal Justice System, October 29, 1987.
10. Bronstein, Testimony.
11. Bronstein, Testimony.
12. *Carmen Harris et al. v. Morris Thigpen, Commissioner, Alabama Department of Corrections.* For more information, contact the ACLU National Prison Project, 1616 P St. NW, #340, Washington, D.C. 20036.

Voices

The authors of this essay are Kathy Boudin, Judy Clark, "D," Katrina Haslip, Maria D.L. Hernandez, Suzanne Kessler, Sonia Perez, Deborah Plunkett, Aida Rivera, Doris Romeo, Carmen Royster, Cathy Salce, Renee Scott, Jenny Serrano, and Pearl Ward.

Introduction

We are writing about ACE because we feel that it has made a tremendous difference in this prison and could make a difference in other prisons. ACE stands for AIDS Counseling and Education. It is a collective effort by women in Bedford Hills Correctional Facility. This article will reflect that collectivity by being a patchwork quilt of many women's voices.

ACE was started by inmates in 1988 because of the crisis that AIDS was creating in our community. According to a blind study done in the Fall-Winter of 1987-88, almost 20 percent of the women entering the New York state prison system were HIV infected.[1] It is likely to be higher today. In addition, women here have family members who are sick and friends who are dying. People have intense fears of transmission through casual contact because we live so closely together. Women are worried about their children and about having safe sex. All this need and energy led to the creation of ACE.

Before ACE

Prior to the formation of ACE, Bedford was an environment of fear, stigma, lack of information, and evasion. AIDS was a word that was whispered. People had no forum in which to talk about their fears. The doctors and nurses showed their biases. They preferred to just give advice, and many wouldn't touch people because of their own fears. There were several deaths. This inflamed people's fear more. People didn't want to look at their own vulnerability—their IV drug use and unsafe sex.

> I felt very negative about people who I knew were sick. To save face, I spoke to them from afar. I felt that they all should be put into a building by themselves because I heard that people who were healthy could make them sick and so they should get specific care. I figured that I have more time (on my sentence); why should I be isolated? They should be. I felt very negative and it came a lot from fear.[2]

Women at Bedford who are sick are housed in a hospital unit called In Patient Care (IPC). ACE members remember what IPC was like before ACE:

> The IPC area—the infirmary—was horrible before, a place where nobody wanted to be. It was a place to go to die. Before ACE people started going there, it looked like a dungeon. It was unsanitary. Just the look of it made people feel like they were going to die. That was the end.

There was no support system for women who wanted to take the HIV-antibody test:

> I had a friend who tested positive. The doctor told her, you are HIV positive, but that doesn't mean you have AIDS. You shouldn't have sex, or have a baby, and you should avoid stress. Period. No information was given to her. No counseling and support. She freaked out.

The Beginning of ACE: Breaking the Silence

Some of us sensed that people needed to talk, but no one would break the silence. Finally, five women got together and made a proposal to the superintendent:

> We said that we ourselves had to help ourselves. We believed that as peers we would be the most effective in education, counseling, and building a community of support. We stated four main goals: to save lives through preventing the spread of HIV; to create more humane conditions for those who are HIV positive; to give support and education to women with fears, questions, and needs related to AIDS; to act as a bridge to community groups to help women as they reenter the community.

The superintendent accepted the proposal. Each of the five women sought out other women in the population who they believed were sensitive and would be interested in breaking the silence. When they reached 35, they stopped and a meeting was called.

Breaking the Silence Changed Us: We Began to Build a Community

At that first meeting a sigh of relief was felt and it rippled out. There was a need from so many directions. People went around the table and said why they were there. About the fourth or fifth woman said, "I'm here because I have AIDS." There was an intense silence. It was the first time anyone had said that aloud in a group. By the end of the meeting, several more women had said that they were HIV positive. Breaking the silence, the faith that it took, and the trust it built was really how ACE started.

Breaking the Silence Meant Something Special to PWAs

I often ask myself how it is that I came to be open about my status. For me, AIDS had been one of my best kept secrets. It took me approximately 15 months to discuss this issue openly. As if not saying it aloud would make it go away. I watched other people with AIDS (PWAs), who were much more open than I was at the time, reveal to audiences their status/their vulnerability, while sharing from a distance, from silence, every word that was being uttered by them. I wanted to be a part of what they were building, what they were doing, their statement, "I am a PWA," because I was. It was a relief when I said it. I could stop going on with the lie. I could be me. People were supportive and they didn't shun me. And now I can go anywhere and be myself.

Breaking the Silence Allowed People to Change Each Other

I was one of those people who once I knew someone had AIDS, I didn't want them around me. That was until Carmen got sick. She was my friend. When I found out she was sick I felt hurt because she didn't have the confidence to tell me. She knew my attitude and didn't want me to turn my back on her. That's when I started researching how you can and can't get the virus and my fear left. ACE also helped me with things I didn't know. Even though Carmen had AIDS and I didn't, I felt that I was living with AIDS through her. I told her that I loved her whether she had AIDS or not.

Breaking the Silence Meant Challenging Stigma

I think there has been a tremendous change in the institution. Before, if people knew about someone, it wasn't to help them, it was only to hurt them. Now people are protective about the people they used to talk about. You will still have people who will use this information as their power, like saying, "You AIDS-ridden this," but you have more people now who will protect those individuals. This is the first time that people in here had something they were doing for other people that they weren't getting something from, some payoff.

Since that beginning two years ago, ACE has gone on to develop a program of work through which we try to reach out to meet the needs of our community.

Supporting PWAs

PWAs and HIV-positive women are at the heart of our work. ACE believes that everyone facing HIV-related illness is confronting issues of life and death and struggling to survive and thrive.

We had to have some place for PWAs to share their experiences with each other. There have been numerous support groups which allowed us to express things that hadn't been verbalized but that had been on our minds. It was interesting to see that we had similar issues: how to tell significant others, our own vulnerability about being open, living with AIDS. My first group was a mixture of people. Some were recently diagnosed and others had been diagnosed for two years. It was informative and it was emotional. Sometimes we would just come to a meeting and cry. Or we might come there and not even talk about the issue of AIDS and just have a humor session because we are just tired of AIDS.

One of the first things that ACE ever did was to work in IPC.

ACE started going to IPC. We painted, cleaned up, made it look so good that now the women want to stay there. We take care of the girls who are sick, making them feel comfortable and alive. Now, women there know they have a friend. They feel free, they talk, and look forward to visits. They know they're not there to die; not like before.

Being a Buddy

I have been involved in ACE for about three years. About a year ago I started visiting the women in IPC. I was really afraid at first. Not afraid of getting sick, but of becoming emotionally involved and then have the women die. At first, I tried to keep my feelings and friendship at a minimum. The more I went, the more I lost this fear. There is one woman I have gotten closer to than the rest. She has been in IPC since I first started going there. We are buddies. For me to be her buddy means unconditionally loving her and accepting her decisions. I go almost every night to IPC. Some nights we just sit there and say nothing. But there is comfort in my presence. She had a stroke before I met her. So there is a lot she cannot do for herself. There are times when I bathe and dress her. Iron her clothes. I do not think of any of these things as chores. Soon she will be going home. I am overjoyed, but I'm also saddened knowing that I will not see her again. I will miss her hugs, her complaining, and her love. But I would do it all over again and I probably will with someone else.

Medical Advocacy

It is obviously a matter of life or death for anyone who is HIV infected to get good medical care and have a good relationship with her health providers. Medical facilities in prisons start out under-staffed and ill equipped, and the AIDS crisis escalated these problems enormously. In the 1970s women prisoners here instituted a class action suit, *Todaro v. Ward,* to demand better medical care. Because of that case, the medical facilities and care at Bedford are monitored for the court by an outside expert. That expert issued a report criticizing all aspects of the medical department for being inade-quately prepared to meet women's AIDS-related medical needs, and the prison faced a court hearing and possible contempt charges. Under that pressure the state agreed to numerous changes that brought new medical staff and resources, including a full-time med-ical director, a part-time infectious disease specialist, and more nurses. ACE was able to institute a medical advocacy plan that allowed ACE members to accompany women to their doctor's consultation visit to insure that nothing was missed. Afterward, there can be a private discussion between the patient and the advocate to clarify matters for the woman, to explore possibilities of treatment, or just to allow the person to express whatever emotions she experienced when she received the news from the doctor.

Peer Education

Our approach is *peer* education, which we believe is best suited for the task of enabling a community to mobilize itself to deal with AIDS. The people doing the training clearly have a personal stake in the community. The education is for all, in the interests of all. This is communicated from the beginning by the women doing the teaching.

Our peer education takes a problem-posing approach. We present issues as problems facing all of us, problems to be examined by drawing on the knowledge and experience of the women being trained. What are the issues between a man and a woman, for example, that make it hard for a woman to demand that her man use a condom? Will distributing free needles or advocating bleach kits stop the spread of AIDS among IV drug users?

Our educational work is holistic. Education is not solely a

presentation of facts, although that is an important part of the trainers' responsibilities. But what impact do feelings and attitudes have on how people deal with facts? Why would a person who knows that you cannot get AIDS by eating from a PWA's plate still act occasionally as if you could? Why would a person who knows that sex without a condom could be inviting death, not use a condom? For education to be a deep process, it involves understanding the whole person; for education to take root within a community, it means thinking about things on a community, social level.

> Coming to prison, living under these conditions, was scary, and AIDS made it even scarier. I was part of a society that made judgments and had preconceived ideas about the women in prison.

Educating Ourselves

Workshops: To become members of ACE, women must be educated through a series of eight workshops. We look at how stigma and blame have been associated with diseases throughout history, and how the sexism of this society impacts on women in the AIDS epidemic. We teach about the nature of the virus, strategies for treatment, and holistic approaches. After the eight weeks, we ask who would like to become involved, and then there is a screening process. The Superintendent has final approval. The workshops are followed by more intensive training of women who become members.

Orientation: When women enter the New York state prison system, they must come first to Bedford Hills, where they either stay or move on after several weeks to one of several other women's prisons. ACE members talk with the women when they first arrive.

> We do orientations of 10 to 35 women. We explain to them how you can and cannot get AIDS, about testing and about ACE. Sometimes the crowd is very boisterous and rude. I say "AIDS" and they don't want to hear about it. But those are the ones I try to reach. After orientation is over, the main ones that didn't want to hear about AIDS are the ones who want to talk more and I feel good about that. A lot of times, their loudness is a defense because they are afraid of their own vulnerability. They know that they are at risk for HIV infection because of previous behaviors. After I finish doing orientation, I have a sense of warmth, because I know I made a difference in some of their lives.

Seminars: One of the main ways we interact with our sisters is through seminars. We talk about AIDS issues with groups of women on living units, in classrooms, and in some of the other prison programs such as family violence, drug treatment, and Children's Center.

> The four back buildings are dormitories, each holding 100 women with double bunked beds. We from ACE gather right after count, with our easel and newsprint and magic markers and our three-by-five cards with the information on whatever presentation we're making. We move in twos and threes through the connecting tunnels to the building. When we arrive some of the women are sitting in the rec room, but many others are in their cubicles/cells. They ask why we're here. We look like a traveling troupe—and we've felt like it, not knowing what to expect. Some women are excited that we're going to talk about AIDS. Others say, "forget it," or "fuck you, I've heard enough about it, it's depressing."

But we begin, and people slowly gather.

> We ask the women to help us role-play a situation such as a woman going home from prison, trying to convince her man, who has been taking care of her while she's inside, to use a condom. Then the role-play is analyzed. What problems are encountered and how do we deal with those problems? We try to come up with suggestions that we can see ourselves using in that situation. We talk about the risk of violence.

One of the most immediate problems people have is whether or not to take the HIV-antibody test. We do not push testing. We explain what the test is and have a group discussion of things the women need to consider. A woman may be inclined to get tested, but she needs to know that she is likely to be transferred upstate before the results come back from the lab. The choice is up to her. Toward the end of the seminar, PWAs talk about their experiences living with AIDS.

> When they speak, they bring together everything that we have said. Not only that, but they let people know that living with AIDS is not instant death. It makes people realize why the struggles, working together, and being as one are so important. When I hear the women who are PWAs speak, it makes me realize that I could have been in their shoes, or I could still be, if they hadn't been willing to talk about their risk behaviors and what has happened to them. It gives me the courage to realize that it's not all about me. It's actually about us.

We end each seminar with all the women standing with our arms around each other or holding hands—without any fear of casual contact—singing our theme song, "Sister."[3] We sing, having come to a new place where we are for each other, unified. We all feel some sense of relief and some sense of hope. Talking about AIDS openly has changed how we live. We leave the seminar with the knowledge that we can talk about AIDS and that we're going to be okay.

Prerelease: This is a program for people within 90 days of going home. They confront the issues of living with AIDS within their prospective communities.

> The women are leaving to go to communities where they are frightened because they don't know if they will find any openness or dialogue. They don't know if they can take the behavior changes they have learned about in here and implement them out there.

The prerelease program also meets the specific needs of PWAs who are leaving the facility. We call this bridging—helping them to connect with follow-up care, assistance, housing. The Bedford community is much more supportive than what most people face when they go outside. During the period before a person is released, she experiences a high level of stress which we have to address on many levels: putting services in place, meeting emotional needs and anxieties, working through issues related to families. We also have to let go, because we become very bonded with each other. There is a weaning process on both ends, and we have to work on preparing both ends of the relationship for this transition.

Although the transition for PWAs may be difficult because of the community of support that ACE has created, it is also true that ACE members come out of Bedford committed and prepared to try to build the same kind of supportive community outside. ACE has created a training ground for women to become community workers in the AIDS crisis.

> ...on the outside I live AIDS through personal experience by having AIDS, and I work at it on a 9 to 5 basis doing case work at Brooklyn AIDS Task Force; come 5 or 6 p.m., that day at the office is over and I am once again all alone. Even though I am involved in other personal AIDS projects, they all lack the closeness that Bedford and ACE provided.

Counseling: When we conduct the seminars and orientation sessions, women come up to us afterward with personal questions and problems. It could be they are HIV positive, or they are thinking of taking the test, or they have a family member who is sick, or they are thinking about getting involved with someone in a relationship.

Sometimes they raise one issue, but underlying it are a lot of other issues they're not yet ready to talk about. Because women know we're in ACE, we're approached in our housing units, at school, on the job, in the mess hall, as we walk from one place to another. Women stop us, needing to talk. We're a haven for women because they know ACE has a principle of confidentiality. Women can trust us not to abuse the information they are sharing with us.

> Peer counseling. I'm just impressed that we can do it. I didn't know what kind of potential we'd have as peers. We talk the language that each of us understands. Even if it's silent, even if it's with our eyes, it's something that each of us seems to understand. I know I wouldn't want someone from the Department of Health who hasn't even taken a Valium to try to educate me about IV drug use. How could they give me helpful hints? I would feel that they are so out of tune with reality that I wouldn't be able to hear them.

AIDS: A Particular Problem for Women

When we begin our workshop on women and AIDS, we ask, "Why are we making a workshop just on how AIDS affects women?" The women come up with a list that answers this question:

- It's a man's world, so AIDS stigmatizes women, such as prostitutes.
- Our dependency on men makes us more vulnerable.
- We have to deal with male cheating and double standards.
- Women are caregivers: responsible for education and health of ourselves, our children, our spouses, and the people we work for.
- Women are isolated and have to deal with all this individually and alone. We need to see it as a social problem so we can act together.
- It's one more strike against Black and Latin women, already suffering from discrimination and racism.

You can't separate AIDS from all of the problems that women face—housing, economics, kids—and the women here, being the most marginalized, face the most problems. ACE tries to draw on women's life experiences to reflect on the problems that we share as women. We believe that by looking at our lives we can get individual strength and also build a social consciousness.

> I was conscious of women before I came in here, but not on that level. ACE has made it deeper. ACE made me realize that AIDS

is bigger than each individual woman, that it's going to take all of us coming together. I never knew so many things affected just women. I had looked at issues as a Black woman—religious issues, being a single parent or not—but I had never reflected on being a woman in society.

A Crisis and Opportunity for Our Community

We are a small community and we are so isolated you can feel it—the suffering, the losses, the fears, the anxiety. Out in the street you don't have a community of women affected and living together facing a problem in this same way. We can draw on the particular strengths that women bring: nurturance, caring, and personal openness. So many women prisoners have worked in nursing and old age homes. Yet when they did, they were never given respect. Here these same activities are valued, and the women are told "thank you," and that creates initiative and feelings of self-worth. And ACE helps us to be more self-conscious about a culture of caring that as women we tend to create in our daily lives.

> For the first time in prison I was part of a group that cared about other prisoners in prison. What did that feel like? It felt like I wasn't alone in caring about people, because in this type of setting I was beginning to wonder about people caring.

Our Impact on Women

We know that we have played a role in communicating information about what is safe and what is not safe in sexual behavior—both between a man and woman and between two women—and we have certainly been able to create open and relaxed discussions about all this. But we know that actually changing behaviors is another leap ahead of us. We are learning that it's not a one-shot deal, that information doesn't equal behavior change, and it's not just an individual thing. Social norms have to change, and this takes time. And when you talk about women having to initiate change you're up against the fact that women don't have that kind of empowerment in this society. Women who have been influenced by ACE have experienced a change in attitude, but it is unclear whether this will translate into behavior change once they leave the prison.

> When I first started taking the workshops I was 100 percent against using condoms. And yet I like anal sex. But now my views are different. We're the bosses of our own bodies. You know, a lot of people say it's a man's world. Well, I can't completely agree.

Our Diversity Is a Strength

We are a diverse community of women: Black, Latin, and white, and also from countries throughout the world. In ACE there was at first a tendency to deny the differences, maybe out of fear of disunity. Now there is a more explicit consciousness growing that we can affirm our diversity and our commonality because both are important. In the last workshop on women, we broke for a while into three groups— Black, Latin, and white women—to explore the ways AIDS impacted on our particular culture and communities. We are doing more of those kinds of discussions and developing materials that address concerns of specific communities. The Hispanic Sector of ACE is particularly active, conducting seminars in Spanish and holding open meetings for the population to foster Hispanic awareness of AIDS issues.

> The workshops didn't deal enough with different ethnic areas, and being Puerto Rican and half-Indian, some things seemed ridiculous in terms of the Hispanic family. Some of the ways people were talking about sex wouldn't work in a traditional Hispanic family. For example, you can't just tell your husband that he has to wear a condom. Or say to him, "You have to take responsibility." These approaches could lead to marital rape or abuse. The empowerment of Hispanic women means making sure that their children are brought up.

Working in a Prison

We have a unique situation at Bedford Hills. We have a prison administration that is supportive of inmates developing a peer-based program to deal with AIDS. However, because we are in a prison there are a lot of constraints and frustrations. Before we had staff persons to supervise us, we could not work out of an office space. That meant that we couldn't see women who wanted to talk on an individual level unless we ran into them in the yard or rec room.

You could be helping someone in IPC take her daily shower; it's taking longer than usual because she is in a lot of pain or she needs to talk, but that's not taken into consideration when the officer tells you that you have to leave immediately because it's "count-time." You could be in the rec room, a large room with a bunch of card tables, loud music, and an officer overseeing groups of women sitting on broken-down chairs. You're talking to a woman in crisis who needs comforting. You reach out to give her a hug and the C.O. may come over to admonish you, "No physical contact, ladies." Or maybe a woman has just tested positive. She's taken her first tentative steps to reach out by talking to someone from ACE and joining a support group. Days after her first meeting, she is transferred to another prison.

It's been difficult to be able to call ourselves counselors and have our work formally acknowledged by the administration. Counseling is usually done by professionals in here because it carries such liability and responsibility. We're struggling for the legitimacy of peer counseling. The reality is that we've been doing it in our daily lives here through informal dialogue. We now have civilian staff to supervise us, and Columbia University will be conducting a certification training program to justify the title "peer counselor."

After working over two years on our own, we are now being funded by a grant from the New York State AIDS Institute, coordinated by Columbia University School of Public Health and by Women and AIDS Resource Network (WARN). The money has allowed hiring staff to work with ACE. ACE began as a totally volunteer inmate organization with no office or materials, operating on a shoestring and scrambling for every meeting. Now we have an office in a prime location of the prison, computers, and a civilian staff responsible for making certain that there is something to show for their salaries. Inmates who used to work whenever they could find the time are now paid 73 cents a day as staff officially assigned to the ACE Center. The crises are no longer centered around the problems of being inside a prison, but more on how to sustain momentum and a real grassroots initiative in the context of a prison. This is a problem faced by many other community organizations when they move past the initial momentum and become more established institutions.

Building a Culture of Survival

When, in the spring of 1987, we said, "Let's make quilt squares for our sisters who have died," there were more than 15 names. Over the next year we made more and more quilt squares. The deaths took a toll not just on those who knew the women but on all of us. Too many women were dying among us. And, for those who were HIV positive or worried that they might be, each death heightened their own vulnerabilities and fears. We have had to develop ways to let people who are sick know that if they die, their lives will be remembered, they will be honored and celebrated, and they will stay in our hearts.

> I remember our first memorial. Several hundred women contributed money—25 cents, 50 cents, a dollar—for flowers. Both Spanish and Black women sang and in the beginning everyone

held hands and sang "That's What Friends Are For," and in the end we sang "Sister." People spoke about what Ro meant to them. Ro had died and we couldn't change that. But we didn't just feel terrible. We felt love and caring and that together we could survive the sadness and loss.

In the streets, funerals were so plastic, but here, people knew that it could be them. It's not just to pay respect. When we sang "Sister," there was a charge between us. Our hands were extended to each other. There was a need for ACE and we could feel it in the air.

It was out of that same need that ACE was formed. It will be out of that same need that ACE will continue to strive to build community and an environment of trust and support. We are all we have—ourselves. If we do not latch on to this hope that has strengthened us and this drive that has broken our silence, we too will suffer and we will remain stigmatized and isolated. Feel our drive in our determination to make changes, and think "community," and make a difference.

Notes

1. Perry F. Smith et al., *Infection Among Women Entering the New York State Correctional System* (1990), unpublished manuscript.
2. All quotations are from the authors' conversations with prisoners at Bedford Hills.
3. By Cris Williamson, from the album *The Changer and the Changed*, Olivia Records, 1975.

Having AIDS and Being Loved

ANONYMOUS

Most of the articles I have been reading I find very depressing for my future. It is terrible to think that because I have AIDS I have to face the rest of my life alone—without a loving companion.

I was diagnosed with AIDS in March of '88. Shortly after that, I was pursuing my present lover, with whom I was working, doing educational work around AIDS. Knowing and teaching the facts about safer sex are one thing; but actually putting them into practice is completely different.

My first reaction to my lover's lack of interest in establishing a relationship with me was, "Is it because I have AIDS?" At that particular time, she couldn't answer me; this only led me to believe that was the true reason. But as months went by, we began enriching our friendship through many talks. We talked of her position on sex. She said she could only feel comfortable venturing into a relationship with me if I promised that I would/could respect her wishes for what she called "Absolutely Safe Sex."

Well, it finally happened—Christmas of '88 to be exact. We started out with the notion of absolutely safe sex, which can create both feelings of total satisfaction but also feelings of wanting more. I must say at this time my lover was and still is interested in exploring the possibilities of using barriers (dental dams and finger cots); but I cannot deal with them. They just emphasize the fact of my disease, and even though I may want to be touched in certain areas, I can't deal with that emphasis of feeling like some *freak!* So I learned to accept that pleasure despite our limitations.

Through attending many talks by professionals, she has changed some of her positions. I always felt that I posed no danger to her by me going down on her—and through months of conversations she has leaned towards the possibilities (few and far between).

But I am patient and accept her struggle of having to feel comfortable in what we do. We also have found ways to kiss without dry kissing but still without deep kissing. There are so many ways of being sensual with your tongue in the area of your mouth without having to stick your tongue inside.

I totally accept her position. We can no longer say we have Absolutely Safe Sex—but the main thing is we together have found ways of making love that are totally acceptable for *US*.

I must add that my lover is an extraordinary person, and I love her for many reasons. And if it wasn't for my persistence and her acceptance, I wouldn't have experienced this wonderful love we've found together.

The *sad* part of all this is I have to leave my lover here in prison—which is devastating for me. I know I will never experience the love I found with her—which is totally unconditional love. Again, I must say she is a *rarity* in society! But I can only look at this from the positive aspect of it all; that is, even though I have AIDS, she has shown me that love is still possible!

To my lover: you have given me something I will cherish for the rest of my life, and no matter when we do part, always know you have made me the happiest person alive! I love you today, always, and forever. You will always be in my heart, even though we must part.

Pregnant Women and HIV

RISA DENENBERG

HIV-positive pregnant women are a focus for some of the most deep-seated value judgments about AIDS. The media's persistent portrayal of a health-failing infant or toddler with AIDS pushes the concept of "innocent" versus "guilty" to the extreme. However, every child born is born of a woman. The majority of women who deliver HIV-infected infants are unaware of their own antibody status until they are faced with health problems in their children.

The Centers for Disease Control (CDC), health providers, politicians, and community leaders have variously suggested routine HIV testing in prenatal clinics, counseling which would encourage women who tested positive to have abortions, and compulsory sterilization of HIV-positive women. Several states have anonymously tested blood samples of newborns for HIV antibodies with the goal of determining perinatal (mother-to-baby) transmission of HIV antibodies (not the virus itself) during pregnancy. Florida and Michigan require HIV testing of pregnant women. Rhode Island allows testing of newborns without maternal consent. Similar laws are now being considered or enacted in other states. The stated goal of such laws and testing programs is usually to find HIV-infected children. This demonstrates a disregard for the woman's well-being, as well as being scientifically incorrect, since the HIV status of newborns cannot be determined by such early testing. Although virtually all children born to HIV-positive mothers receive their mothers' antibodies and will test positive, not all are actually infected with the virus. An uninfected child may retain the mother's antibodies for 15 to 18 months, but will eventually test negative.

If you scratch the surface, the typical obstetrician, pediatrician, legislator, health administrator, or next door neighbor probably favors coercive methods that would prevent the "tragedy and cost" of

HIV-infected children. These "methods" represent a value of fetus over woman. These views, and the public policies that follow, further constrict the already narrowed scope of freedom of HIV-positive women. Testing during pregnancy or immediately after delivery puts a woman at risk of losing certain rights without any promise of treatment or services. She may fear loss of custody of her children, or pressure to abort or accept sterilization. These are not unfounded fears.

The history of coercive policies and laws regarding reproduction is noteworthy. Laws against abortion have resulted in enormous increases in maternal deaths. In the 1930s, 27 U.S. states had compulsory sterilization laws for the "unfit." Medical policies have resulted in very high sterilization rates for Native American, Puerto Rican, and poor women.

At present we have only broad estimates regarding transmission rates of HIV from woman to fetus during pregnancy, ranging from 20 to 50 percent. The course of HIV illness is different in women than in men, and it is different in children than in adults. Not enough is known at this time to provide comprehensive advice or counseling to HIV-positive women. Even as we learn more, the rights of these women demand scrupulous protection. No situation has called more loudly for a feminist response.

Effect of Pregnancy on the HIV-Positive Woman and the Fetus She Carries

It is best in many respects to view the woman and her fetus as a unit during pregnancy. Simply stated, and with a few important exceptions, what is good for the woman is good for the fetus, and what is bad for the woman is bad for the fetus.

Some things make it more difficult to say with any degree of certainty how HIV-positive mothers or their babies will fare or are faring now. Few studies exist. Most have been conducted retrospectively, often after the woman has died of AIDS, or on groups of women identified because their children became sick. This way of studying phenomena can distort the actual experience. Some important data are never retrieved or considered. Women and children who do well medically are often rendered invisible by this type of research. For example, researchers initially believed that all or most children born of HIV-positive women would develop AIDS and that pregnancy would accelerate the course of HIV disease. Retrospective studies seemed to confirm their predictions, but current data do not support either notion. Still, it is clear that not enough is known.

Additionally, many variables cannot be separated from a

woman's HIV status. Sexually transmitted infections (STDs) have increased dramatically, especially since the development of nonbarrier methods of birth control. STDs alone account for a significant number of complications and deaths in pregnant women and for problems for the fetus. Herpes, syphilis, gonorrhea, and chlamydia, to name only a few, have dramatically increased during the years since AIDS was first observed. The use of prescription and street drugs, alcohol, and tobacco are all known to affect the outcome of pregnancy for both mother and baby. Several of these habits may exist in an HIV-positive woman, and it can be difficult to sort out what is causing what.

In fact, many HIV-positive woman are intravenous drug users (IVDUs), and most studies done on HIV-positive women are done on IVDUs or former IVDUs enrolled in methadone programs. A myth exists that IVDUs may not be able to get pregnant; drug use and related medical problems may result in irregular periods, but this is not the same as infertility. This myth, combined with the social and economic realities of drug use, may account for research findings that IVDUs are less likely to use contraceptives. So these women may be at greater risk for both pregnancy and infection.

Pregnancy may afford a woman the motivation to take better care of herself. During a pregnancy, a woman is less likely to shoot drugs, smoke cigarettes, or drink alcohol, and more likely to eat well. She may feel better about herself and get more approval from others. These are important factors in making a decision about carrying a pregnancy, as well as in the relatively favorable outcomes seen in HIV-positive, asymptomatic women.

Basically, the best data available from the limited research studies point to the following likely trends. This summary should be considered an interpretation of these studies. Obviously, much more well-designed research is needed and may outdate these statements.

- Asymptomatic HIV-positive women get pregnant at essentially the same rate as HIV-negative women. In other words, fertility is not affected by HIV infection.
- Asymptomatic HIV-positive women appear to have no more risk of poor outcomes in pregnancy than other similar women. A "poor pregnancy outcome" (a technical term) is used here to refer to the variations from a normal course of pregnancy, such as premature deliveries, small babies, miscarriages, stillbirths, and so on.
- Worsening of HIV disease does not seem to occur more rapidly during pregnancy in asymptomatic women. There is no present

evidence that pregnancy will cause an asymptomatic woman to become symptomatic.

- Women with advanced ARC or AIDS are likely to get sicker more quickly if they carry a pregnancy to term.
- Estimates of rates of transmission of HIV from mother to fetus range from 20 to 50 percent.
- There is some risk of HIV transmission through breast-feeding, but it is probably a small risk.
- There is no reason to choose C-section over vaginal delivery simply because a woman is HIV positive. [See endnotes 1-12 for background and research that supports these assertions.]

Key Issues in Decision Making

More than 70 percent of women who are HIV positive are poor, urban-dwelling women of color. HIV transmission is generally due to IV drug use or heterosexual intercourse with a man who is an IVDU. Janet Mitchell, a Black obstetrician/gynecologist who works at Harlem Hospital in New York City caring for women with "high-risk" pregnancies, describes such women aptly: "They are survivors. They are smart. In a world that denies their existence they struggle for some sense of self. Oftentimes that sense of self is intimately related to their ability to procreate and mother."[13]

The decision to carry a pregnancy to term, or to have an abortion, exists presently in a highly charged political atmosphere. For an HIV-positive woman the decision is complicated by an uncertain future for both the woman and the children she bears. But poor women are accustomed to taking risks, and to struggling against uncertain odds. It should not be surprising that studies reveal that a woman's knowledge of being HIV positive is not associated with her choosing an abortion.[14-16] Other concerns may have a higher priority, or abortion may not even be available. The Hyde Amendment, enacted in 1977, denies women who receive Medicaid access to federal funds for abortion services. At present, only nine states and the District of Columbia fund abortions on the basis of a woman's choice. Since many poor women obtain medical services only through Medicaid (or, if ineligible for Medicaid, not at all), they do not have the option to terminate a pregnancy. In addition, some abortion facilities refuse to provide the service to a woman who admits to being HIV positive.

Since current knowledge suggests that in early HIV infection a woman and her fetus both have a reasonable chance of doing well, how can a policy of advising such women to abort, delay, or forgo pregnancy be justified?

Another decision a pregnant HIV-positive woman faces is breast-feeding. The risk of transmission from breast milk is likely to be less than the risk of transmission during pregnancy. HIV is found in breast milk in similar concentration to saliva, but since much more is ingested and the infant's digestive system is immature, the risk is likely to be greater than the extremely low risk from kissing. A study of women in a Lusaka, Zambia, teaching hospital observed that children can acquire HIV solely from breast-feeding.[17] In the United States, a positive woman would probably be advised by laypersons and health providers not to breast-feed. But positive women in Zambia are not discouraged from breast-feeding their children. One explanation offered is that these children were at a greater risk of illness from formula feeding, which is associated with life-threatening diarrhea in nonindustrialized countries because it is often diluted with unsterilized water. Many questions are raised when medical advice is in conflict in different populations.

Given the paucity of information currently available, the only acceptable counseling to pregnant women on these and other questions of such a personal nature would be full explanations of the available information, a nondirective approach, and complete medical and social support for the woman's decision.

Notes

1. P. A. Selwyn et al., "Prospective Study of Human Immunodeficiency Virus Infection and Pregnancy Outcomes in Intravenous Drug Use," Journal of the American Medical Association (JAMA), Vol. 261, no. 9, 1989, pp. 1,289-1,294.
2. H. L. Minkoff, "Care of Pregnant Women Infected with Human Immunodeficiency Virus," JAMA, Vol. 258, no. 19, 1987, pp. 2,714-2,717.
3. J. Gloeb, "Human Immunodeficiency Virus Infection in Women: The Effects of Human Immunodeficiency Virus on Pregnancy," American Journal of Obstetrics and Gynecology, Vol. 159, no. 3, 1988, pp. 756-761.
4. "HIV Infection: Obstetric and Perinatal Issues," Lancet, April 9, 1988, pp. 806-807.
5. L. M. Koonin et al., "Pregnancy-associated Deaths Due to AIDS in the United States," JAMA, Vol. 261, no. 9, 1989, pp. 1,306-1,309.
6. European Collaborative Study, "Mother-to-Child Transmission of HIV Infection," Lancet, November 5, 1988, pp. 1,039-1,043.
7. R. Bayer, JAMA, Vol. 261, no. 7, 1989, p. 993.
8. R. Hoff et al., "Seroprevalence of Human Immunodeficiency Virus Among Childbearing Women," New England Journal of Medicine, Vol. 318, March 3, 1988, pp. 525-529.
9. H. Minkoff et al., "Pregnancies Resulting in Infants with Acquired Immune Deficiency Syndrome or AIDS-Related Complex: Follow-up of Mothers, Children and Subsequent Born Siblings," Obstetrics and Gyne-

cology, Vol. 69, 1987, pp. 288-291.
10. L. R. Callum et al., "Does Pregnancy Influence Disease Progression in HIV Antibody Positive Women?" Presented at European Conference on Clinical Aspects of HIV Infection, Brussels, December 10-11, 1987.
11. S. Landesman et al., "Serosurvey of Human Immunodeficiency Virus in Parturients," _JAMA,_ Vol. 258, no. 19, 1987, pp. 2,701-2,703.
12. E. Schoenbaum et al., "The Effect of Pregnancy on Progression of HIV-Related Disease," New York City HIV Perinatal Transmission Collaborative Study, Montefiore Medical Center, Albert Einstein College of Medicine, New York City, 1989.
13. Janet Mitchell, "What About the Mothers of HIV Infected Babies? National AIDS Network Multicultural Notes on AIDS," _Education & Service,_ Vol. 1, no. 10, April 1988.
14. P. A. Selwyn et al., "Knowledge of HIV Antibody Status and Decisions to Continue or Terminate Pregnancy Among Intravenous Drug Users," _JAMA,_ Vol. 261, no. 24, 1989, pp. 3,567-3,571.
15. A. Wiznia et al., "Factors Influencing Maternal Decision Making Regarding Pregnancy Outcome in HIV Infected Women," Albert Einstein College of Medicine, Bronx, NY, _V International Conference on AIDS,_ 1989.
16. M. Barbacci, "Knowledge of HIV Serostatus and Pregnancy Decisions," Johns Hopkins University, Baltimore, MD, _V International Conference on AIDS,_ 1989.
17. S. Hira et al., "Breast-feeding and HIV-1 Transmission," University Teaching Hospital, Lusaka, Zambia, _V International Conference on AIDS,_ 1989.

Mothers and Children

JUDITH WALKER

Most women with AIDS (not to mention those with HIV illnesses not officially recognized as AIDS) are mothers. Unofficial estimates range from "over 50 percent" (New York City Health Department epidemiologist) to "99 percent" (New York City social worker). Yet neither the Centers for Disease Control (CDC), whose statistics are used to plan HIV services nationwide, nor the government of the city with the country's largest number of AIDS cases, records this central piece of information.

The government's indifference toward the actual lives of affected women helps explain the fact that women with AIDS die as much as six times faster after diagnosis than do men. Although more funds must be made available for health care and support services, not all the system's problems come from lack of money. Some come from a failure to care or plan—especially when those in need are female, poor, and, often, people of color.

To some, the official number of children with AIDS may not be frightening. Through April 1990, according to the CDC, there had been a total of 2,258 cases nationwide since the beginning of the epidemic.[1] But there are two problems with this number. First, it is certainly too low (there is an epidemic of undercounting of pediatric HIV infection). In New York City, an informal survey by a branch of the Health Department found 1,300 children living with HIV disease in September 1989, while the same agency's official AIDS Surveillance Unit counted only 221: less than a fifth as many. Apparently there is a lack of will in the government to confront the true extent of pediatric AIDS. Could it be that the necessary services would cost too much? Or that somebody—the government? the taxpayers?—does not consider these particular babies worth the cost?

The other problem is that the pediatric AIDS cases that we have today are just the tip of the iceberg. Based on current estimates of HIV infection in New York City alone, which range from 200,000 to 400,000, with women now making up about 13 percent of all cases, there are probably at least 26,000 HIV-positive women of childbearing age. The CDC estimates that one million Americans—probably including over 100,000 women—are infected. And virtually no planning or allocating of funds is taking place to meet the health care needs of those women and their children.

Fragmented Service Delivery

HIV illness is a family disease. Most mothers of children with HIV disease are themselves positive; many are ill. But, too often, services for mothers and children are not only inadequate, but divided among multiple agencies, each with its own regulations, visits, and paperwork. If there are adolescents in the family, still more agencies can be involved. Sometimes the result might be ludicrous, if it did not have tragic effects on real families, as in the case of the Carreros (not their real name) in the Bronx, who had to put up with a *child* care worker sent by one agency, who would make lunch for the children but not the mother, and a *home* care worker sent by another agency, who would make lunch for the mother but not the children, bumping into each other and everyone else every day. Can this approach to providing services possibly be explained as cost effective?

Substandard Care

Most mothers and children with HIV illnesses are uninsured or are Medicaid insured, meaning, in general, that they receive inadequate health care. In New York City, most of them get their primary health care from the emergency rooms of the already crippled municipal hospital system. Patients who have been admitted to these hospitals may wait for 24 hours in the emergency room before receiving a bed. Fifteen percent of funded nursing jobs, and up to twice as many of the lab technician or social worker jobs, go unfilled because of the bad working conditions and low pay in these municipal hospitals.

In June 1989, a municipal hospital with New York City's highest rate of AIDS cases per capita (Kings County Hospital), still did not offer aerosol pentamadine, which by then was regularly used in better endowed hospitals to prevent PCP, the leading killer of PWAs. Although the drug had been front-page news in newspapers and medical bulletins, the hospital director, James Buford, told activists that he had never heard of the drug.

Emergency rooms do not as a rule offer continuity of care: patients usually see a different doctor at each visit (and it is not uncommon for patients to go from hospital to hospital as well, often giving false names, in order to avoid detection by the government—if they lack green cards or social security numbers—or even by their own families). For HIV patients, because of the nature of the disease, this lack of continuity is very dangerous.

The condition of a given PWA varies widely, including times when she feels fine, times when she is symptomatic but self-sufficient, times when she needs medical care at home, and times when she needs to be hospitalized. But Medicaid does not recognize this changing reality; it will not cover the cost of home-based health care, even though as a result PWAs must stay unnecessarily in hospitals at a far greater cost to the government.

Inadequate Support Services

Too often being a mother with HIV illness means confronting how little the government and the health care system care about your well-being. It can mean an unbearable burden on top of problems like addiction or homelessness that you are also not receiving help with. It can mean lacking basic information about how to get help. It can mean having to choose between taking care of yourself and taking care of a sick child, husband, or companion, because you do not have the strength or the support to do both, and because the government, if it finds you have been hospitalized, is likely to remove your children and put them in foster care. It can mean lacking the resources—such as child care or transportation—that would make it possible for you to get treatment that could save your life—treatment that *is* saving the lives of other people who don't have children to take care of. It can mean being poorly cared for in your own home by health care workers who are overworked, underpaid, and undertrained. It can mean agonizing about what will happen to your children after you die, without the legal or psychological counsel for either you or them, and it can mean dying without any security that at least provisions will be made to keep your children together.

These examples do not reflect on our health and welfare systems alone, but more fundamentally on a wealthy society that does not really believe poor people are entitled to adequate health care, humane living conditions, or decent jobs.

Treatment Issues for Children

Pharmaceutical company greed, government inaction, bureaucratic red tape, and the inability of children to fight for themselves have resulted in a major failure to develop effective pediatric AIDS treatments.

Clinical trials, in which promising new drugs are studied in actual patients, have been a major source of free, up-to-date treatment for adult PWAs, but they do not serve children well. The development of AIDS treatments for children lags far behind the process for adults. It was not until spring 1990 that the FDA finally approved AZT for children, three years after its approval for adults. So far it is the only fully approved treatment for HIV-positive children. Pharmaceutical companies do not invest in testing pediatric AIDS treatments because children are not a "big enough market," and the government does not want to pick up the bill either. There is a major research gap.

According to the AIDS Clinical Trials Information Service of the Public Health Service (ACTIS), which lists all government-sponsored trials and many independent ones, six drugs were being tested for pediatric HIV infection in a total of 290 open and closed trials in June 1989. ACTIS lists 225 trials of 84 different drugs for adults.

The government requires new drugs to be tested differently and more cautiously in children because children's systems are different and more vulnerable. Unfortunately, a result of this appropriate caution is that the victories of AIDS activists in getting new drugs developed and released have not benefited children. In addition, HIV infection in children shows up differently than in adults. Children get different opportunistic infections; HIV affects their brains differently. If there are to be better pediatric AIDS treatments, ways must be found for children to have both increased access to the benefits of adult AIDS research and more research directed to their own unique medical conditions.

Now that AZT *has* been approved, will it reach the uninsured and Medicaid-insured children who make up the bulk of pediatric AIDS cases? Burroughs-Wellcome, the maker of AZT, got front-page publicity in *The New York Times* in October 1989 for volunteering to distribute the drug free of charge to all children in need as an investigational new drug. As of March 1990, only 15 of 180 eligible children at New York's Kings County Hospital were receiving the drug, due to the company's distribution regulations (doctors must see the children twice a week), combined with hospital understaffing. This is probably typical of public hospitals around the country.

Parents and caretakers of children with HIV infection must overcome their tendency to trust the experts to decide what is best for the child. For example, in the Burroughs-Wellcome AZT distribution plan, children are not benefiting from recent medical evidence that, together with pressure by activists, persuaded the FDA to lower the recommended dosage of the drug by 50 percent. This is vital because AZT is highly toxic, causing such serious side effects that many adults could not tolerate it. It is just as effective at half-dosage, with fewer side effects. Under the Burroughs-Wellcome plan, doctors who opt to give children the lower dosage will not receive free medication. Thus, these children are virtually barred from receiving the current standard of AZT treatment.

Many treatments for HIV disease are risky or have serious side effects, but, as with people with cancer who undergo chemotherapy, PWAs are often willing to take the risks. It is difficult to rationalize subjecting children (usually children do not make their own treatment decisions) to some of these treatments unless it is absolutely necessary. But currently there is no way to tell whether an infant has the virus and thus needs treatment. Fifty to 80 percent of children born with HIV antibodies lose them by the age of 15 months and are totally virus free. As a result, toxic drugs like AZT are being tested on infants who are not necessarily at risk of developing AIDS. If a method of diagnosing HIV infection in infants is found, it is crucial that it be made available to all infants. In the absence of a reliable diagnosis, parents and caretakers of infants must be fully informed— or must inform themselves—of the possible risks and benefits of all trials and treatments.

There is a drug called Bactrim that has been on the market for years, in common use as a treatment for both serious and minor infections in children and adults. During the AIDS crisis, it was found that Bactrim also works well to prevent PCP in adults with HIV disease.

In Miami, which has the nation's second highest concentration of pediatric AIDS, doctors also use Bactrim to prevent PCP in HIV-positive children. There, only 10 percent of infected children develop PCP. In New York City, Bactrim is not used for this purpose; 43 percent of infected children get PCP.[2] Hundreds of kids have been harmed, often fatally, by bouts of pneumonia that could have been prevented.

The explanation for this is bureaucratic. Developed before the AIDS crisis, Bactrim is not officially listed as a PCP prophylactic (preventative drug). For doctors to prescribe a drug for a non-recommended use involves a certain amount of risk. Apparently Miami doctors are willing to take this risk. The government also has not been willing to spend money to notify doctors that Bactrim is now officially recognized as a PCP prophylactic. In late 1989, NIAID

(National Institute of Allergy and Infectious Diseases) announced its *intention* to recommend widespread use of Bactrim for children, but the recommendation would not be available in the privately published "Red Book" (the bible of pediatric medical care)[3] for a year. How many children have gotten PCP during that year? This is a typical example of how the bureaucracy drags its heels while people die.

Children Without Parents

AIDS strikes many people in the childbearing years. The epidemic is producing thousands of orphans and foster children. Even those who are not HIV positive are stigmatized by having had parents with AIDS.

In New York City alone, estimates of "AIDS orphans" run from 20,000 by 1995 (New York City Health Department)[4] to between 75,000 and 85,000 by the end of the decade (the Panos Institute; the figures refer to uninfected children only).[5]

Because of a shortage of foster homes, many of these children are already being placed in group homes that some experts fear will become as large and bleak as the orphanages of the past.

Social workers and media horror stories tell of hospital wards filled with "AIDS babies." An AIDS professional in Brooklyn tells of a child orphaned by AIDS whose relatives refused to take him; luckily, his nurse and her husband adopted him. How many children can hope to be so fortunate?

Children as "Victims"

We have all watched conservative politicians preach about the "right to life" of the fetus while slashing government programs for children (not to mention prenatal care that would lower the shocking infant mortality rate in the United States). In the same way, society speaks of "innocent" children with AIDS—as contrasted with "guilty" adults who "chose" to get sick—while failing to provide anything like adequate services for them. This is hypocrisy.

Adults with HIV disease have to battle the medical and social service establishments every step of the way to get new drugs developed and made accessible, to stop discrimination, and to avoid being written off as doomed victims. Infants and children are not equipped for these battles. Children with HIV illnesses are *expected* to die young, and this gives politicians an excuse not to fund programs to help them. The victim language must stop.

Social Issues

The stigma of AIDS is a painful reality. For the mother, it frequently means rejection by friends, mate, or family. If she has an HIV-positive child, it can mean being treated as if she is solely responsible for her child's illness (as if men did not play a role in HIV transmission).

For children, HIV infection can be cause for the cruelest discrimination. Local school districts have sued to bar children with AIDS from attending school. In New York City, due to nonenforcement of anti-discrimination policies, de facto discrimination against HIV-infected children in hospitals and day care centers is common. Even HIV-negative children who are from countries such as Haiti, which has been inaccurately portrayed as having a higher rate of AIDS, or gay adolescents, are often stigmatized and experience the cruelty of strangers.

Demands

- Family-centered case management for mothers and children with HIV infection.
- More primary care for low-income women and children.
- Medicaid coverage of home care for PWAs.
- Residential drug treatment for mothers, pregnant women, and their children.
- Support services for mothers with AIDS.
- Nontraditional foster homes.
- Humane treatment of survivors and "AIDS orphans."
- Decent pay, support, and training for health care workers.
- More clinical trials for children.

Acknowledgments

Special thanks to David Kirschenbaum of ACT UP, Emily Gordon, and Suki Ports for their help with this essay.

Notes

1. Centers for Disease Control, *HIV/AIDS Surveillance Report,* December 1989.
2. Personal communication with David Kirschenbaum.
3. *Pediatric Red Book,* Academy of Pediatrics, 1990.
4. Bruce Lambert, "AIDS Legacy: A Growing Generation of Orphans," *The New York Times,* July 17, 1989, quoting New York Health Department official Dr. Pauline Thomas.
5. Panos Institute, in association with Save the Children Society of Denmark, New Zealand, Sweden, and the U.K.: "AIDS and Children—a Family Disease," November 1989.

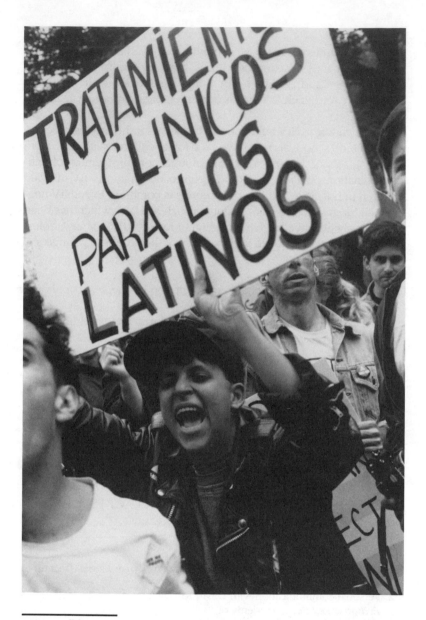

Activists call for treatment facilities in Latino communities when ACT UP storms the National Institutes of Health in Bethesda, Maryland, May 21, 1990.

Photo by Jocelyn Taylor

No Puedo Confiar en Nadie
(I Can't Trust Anyone)

ANONIMO (ANONYMOUS)

No voy a decirles mi nombre puesto que en esta corta historia los nombres no cuentan. Soy hispana y tengo hijos y tuve un esposo por el cual fuí infectada. Cuando yo me enteré de la enfermedad de mi esposo lo único que pensé fue en ayudarlo y darle todo mi apoyo, pero él empezó a decaer, puesto que aparte de tener el SIDA él bebía continuamente y la situación familiar en vez de estar más unida se hacía cada vez más imposible. Mi esposo llegaba bebido y me maltrataba y yo me negaba en abandonarlo puesto que pensaba que él me necesitaba. Yo sentía que el peso familiar recaía sobre mí y trataba lo más posible por ocultarles a mis hijos la realidad de nuestras vidas.

Después vino lo peor para mí cuando me dijeron que yo estaba infectada por el mortal virus. ¡Que desgracia Dios mío! Cómo seguir adelante, qué desesperación sentí, no porque tuviera miedo a morir, sino porque tenía miedo por mis hijos; quién se iba a ser cargo de ellos y a darles todo el amor que unas criaturas pequeñas necesitan. Cómo explicarles a mis hijos que muy pronto su padre iba a morir y que tal vez muy pronto su madre también los iba a dejar.

Se me hacía tan difícil seguir luchando, aparte de que tenía y sigo teniendo miedo a confiar en las personas ajenas a mi desgracia.

No puedo olvidar que donde yo vivía antes de venir a Nueva York tenía amistades que yo creía sinceras y pensar que esas mismas gentes cuando supieron de mi desgracia en vez de ayudarme y darme apoyo lo que hicieron fue pasar mi nombre por el radio y la historia de lo que pasaba en mi familia. Los vecinos quisieron quemar mi casa, y nadie quiso comprar mis muebles y pertenencias que yo estaba vendiendo para tener dinero para el viaje. Por eso yo no puedo confiar en nadie y se me hace muy difícil creer en la bondad de este mundo.

Fueron muy pocas las personas que me ayudaron. Desde que mi esposo murió dejándome con esta terrible enfermedad, yo he tenido que darme fuerzas y aliento para no dejarme vencer por la enfermedad y la depresión. Trato de pensar lo menos posible que lo tengo y tal vez, porque tengo fé y esperanza en una cura, puedo gozar de mis hijos y darles lo mejor de mí. Porque no quiero que pase lo que pasó donde yo vivía antes, trato de protejer a mis hijos de la maldad de la gente que solo piensa en causar mas daño sin pensar por lo que uno está pasando. Y porque trato de proterjerlos me encierro en el mundo que yo he formado con mis hijos y trato de no hacer amistad con nuevas gentes porque les tengo desconfianza y porque pienso que son muy pocas las personas aparte de las amistades que tengo, que son pocas, que entenderían y me aceptarían sin tener miedo de mí.

Es muy triste llegar a la conclusión que la única forma de ser un poco feliz es encenrándome en mi mundo. Porque el mundo de afuera es un mundo hostil que lo único que piensa es en condenar, y viven faltos de bondad para con el que está en desgracia.

Ahora vivo feliz a mi manera. Encontré un trabajo y eso me ayuda a darles un poco de seguridad material a mis hijos que son lo más importante para mí.

Trato de que mis hijos nunca me vean llorar mi pena. Digo que vivo feliz porque solo en su inocencia y amor de hijos encuentro amor sincero, y eso para mí es lo que me hace luchar y seguir adelante. Aunque a veces me derrumbo y lloro sola mi desgracia siento que es mejor así, vivir sin amistades a tener que vivir en la zozobra de si puedes o no puedes confiar plenamente en ellas.

I won't mention my name because in this short account names don't matter. I'm Hispanic and I have children and I had a husband by whom I was infected. When I found out about his sickness, I could think only about helping him and giving him all my support, but he began to deteriorate. Besides having AIDS, he was drinking continually, and the family situation, instead of becoming more united, became more and more difficult. My husband would come home drunk and beat me up, but I couldn't think of leaving him because I thought he needed me. I felt that the burden of keeping the family together was on my shoulders, and I tried my best to hide the real situation from my children.

Then came the worst for me when they told me that I had the

deadly virus. My God, what a tragedy! How could I go on? The desperation I felt was not because I was afraid to die but because I was afraid there would be no one to take care of my children. How could I explain to them that soon their father would die and maybe their mother would leave them soon too?

It was so hard to keep struggling, besides the fact that I have been so afraid to confide in anyone about my terrible condition.

I can't forget about where I came from before I came to New York. I had friends I thought were sincere, but these same people, when they learned of my situation, instead of helping me and giving me support, they put my name and the story of what happened to my family on the radio. The neighbors wanted to burn down my house, and no one would buy the furniture and belongings I was selling to have money for my trip. That's why I can't trust anyone or believe that there's goodness in the world.

There were very few people who helped me. Since my husband died, leaving me with this terrible sickness, I've had to have strength and courage so I won't be defeated by the sickness and the depression. I try to think as little as possible about what I have, and maybe, because I have faith and hope that there might be a cure, I can enjoy my children and give them the best that I have. Because I don't want what happened where I lived before to happen again, I try to protect my children from the evil of other people who only think of doing more harm without thinking about what a person might be going through. I stay enclosed in the world I have created with my children and try not to make new friends because I don't trust anyone except for the few friends I have who understand me and accept me without being afraid.

It's sad to realize that the only way to be even a little happy is to just stay in my own world. The outside world is hostile and people only think of judging—living without compassion for someone in my condition.

I'm happy now in my own way. I found a job, and this gives me some material security for my children, who are the most important things in the world to me.

I try never to let my children see my suffering. I say I am happy because it is only in the innocence and love of children that I can find genuine love, and that is why I keep fighting—although sometimes I get depressed and go off alone and cry. I think it is better that way—to live without friends rather than live not knowing whether or not you can trust someone.

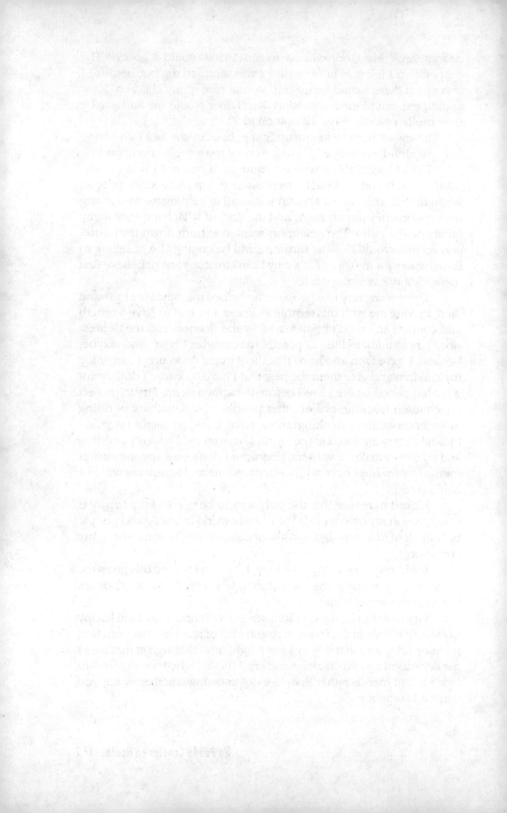

Prostitution and HIV Infection

ZOE LEONARD

POLLY THISTLETHWAITE

> There is existing a moral pestilence which creeps insidiously
> into the privacy of the domestic circle, and draws thence the
> myriads of its victims, and which saps the foundation of that holy
> confidence, the first, most beautiful attraction of home.
>
> W.W. Sanger, M.D., *History of Prostitution*, 1895

Laws prohibiting prostitution and the related "offenses" of so-licitation and loitering have been formed from the rhetoric in struggle "to uphold the nation's morality" or to guard "the family against vice and depravity" or to protect the unsuspecting "general population" from disease. Sometimes prostitution laws are justified in liberal terms; for example, to protect prostitute "victims" from the violence bred by a sexist society. Regardless of legal intent or means of justification, laws prohibiting nonviolent sexual behavior between consenting people violate individual freedom. They cut right through us. With these laws, the state assumes enormous power over our sexualities, our identities, and our lives. The state could use this power to persecute all of us, but instead invokes it discriminatingly to penalize only a select minority.

> A prostitute is said to be one who commits common indiscrim-inate sexual activity for hire, in distinction from sexual activity confined exclusively to one person; therefore a woman who indulges in illicit sexual intercourse with only one man has been said not to be a prostitute. On the other hand, it has been held, whether a woman is a common prostitute does not depend alone upon the number of persons with whom she has illicit intercourse but rather may be judged from all the surrounding circumstances, including her acts, conduct, and utterances, and a determination as to whether she was lacking in discrimination within the commonly accepted meaning of that word in submit-ting to, or offering her body for, illicit sexual intercourse. Since

the usual motive for indiscriminate sexual intercourse is the money paid therefor, prostitution is sometimes defined to be indiscriminate sexual commerce for gain, or for a fee, and gain has been made an element of the crime by statute in some jurisdictions...

Irwin J. Shiffres, J.D., "Prostitution,"
American Jurisprudence, 2nd ed., 1984

Prostitution is illegal in all the United States except in a few counties in Nevada where it is legal and regulated.[1] Criminal definitions of prostitution are sexist, vague, and arbitrarily enforced and applied, as this excerpt from a popular legal text suggests. Early state and municipal legislation defined and prohibited specific sexual acts as prostitution, but this approach proved too difficult to enforce. As a result, legislation over the past 30 years or so has supplemented earlier laws prohibiting not only the sex defined as prostitution, but also the solicitation and loitering behavior determined to precede it. This approach, of course, allows the state more power to arrest and prosecute. The U.S. government spends an estimated $227 million per year on arrests, prosecution, and incarceration of sex workers.[2]

There are many different ways to work as a prostitute. The most visible and recognizable involves street solicitation, but street work constitutes only 10 to 20 percent of prostitution in the United States.[3] Streetwalkers usually make less money and work under more dangerous and stressful conditions than women working as kept mistresses or in brothels, massage parlors, or escort agencies. Racism, ageism, and economic violence dictate that more women of color, poor women, and young women in the sex industry tend to work in disproportionate numbers on the street and, generally, under more unfavorable conditions.

Prostitute arrests and prosecution practices reflect legal discrimination on the basis of gender, race, and class. Of 126,500 people arrested on prostitution charges in 1983, only 10 percent were male heterosexual customers, while 73 percent were female sex workers, and 17 percent were male transvestite or preoperation transsexual workers. Almost 90 percent of prostitutes arrested are women who work the street. Though approximately 50 percent of street prostitutes are women of color, 55 percent of those arrested and 85 percent who actually do jail time are women of color.[4]

Women on the street are more likely to be substance users and are more likely to have sexual partners who are addicted to drugs. High seroprevalence rates reported among street workers have run parallel with reported practice of IV drug use (which assumes unsafe needle sharing) and unprotected sex with IV drug-using men.[5] In addition, some women who may or may not think of themselves as sex workers exchange sex for drugs, especially crack, in desperate situations. Many women believe that only other so-called bad women, whores, and drug users get AIDS. The madonna/whore dichotomy pervades our culture and psyches, making it difficult for many women to make an objective assessment of risk for HIV infection.

Prostitutes as Scapegoats

A German bullet is cleaner than a whore.

Colonel Care Poster, World War I
hygiene propaganda, c. 1918

Along with gay and bisexual men and IVDUs, prostitutes have been blamed for AIDS. Prostitutes have been depicted as "pools of contagion," "reservoirs of infection," and "vectors of transmission" who are "selling death" to the supposedly pure, innocent heterosexual population.

To date, the scientific community's interest in prostitutes has stemmed from the perceived threat of infection posed to straight men. Proposals for mandatory HIV testing for prostitutes have gained popularity in response to these fears, not to concerns about prostitutes' health. Rarely is it suggested that a sex worker test her HIV status in order to seek treatment or to better govern her own life. There has been no real cry of concern for prostitutes' lives, even though female sex workers are at far greater risk of contracting HIV from clients than clients are of contracting HIV from sex workers.[6] In the United States, male-to-female HIV transmission through penis-vagina and penis-oral sex is far more likely than female-to-male transmission.

Most professional sex workers routinely use condoms for both oral and vaginal sex,[7] sometimes by sneaking them on unbeknownst to johns. Sex workers are far more likely to practice safe sex than other sexually active women.[8] But there are barriers to routine condom use. Condoms themselves can be expensive, and not all women can afford them all the time. And like other heterosexual men who prefer not to use condoms, johns will sometimes either refuse to use a condom or will offer more money for skin-to-skin contact. Heterosexual men have a legacy of bearing no responsibility for preventing pregnancy or STD transmission, so it is unusual for johns who do not perceive themselves at risk for AIDS to take responsibility for safe sex with prostitutes. Sex workers may also be at risk for HIV infection from their lovers. Women who use condoms on the job might not—as a way of expressing love or trust or to separate sex for work from sex for pleasure—use barrier methods at home with their lovers. And finally, in many cities, police undermine sex workers' efforts to practice safe sex by confiscating or destroying condoms and bleach during prostitute arrests. In San Francisco, COYOTE (Call Off Your Old Tired Ethics), the prostitutes' advocacy organization, fought this practice and obtained a special order from the police department stopping seizure of condoms and bleach.

Prostitute Seroprevalence Studies

Many studies have been done to determine the rates of HIV infection among women sex workers in the United States, with seroprevalence rates ranging from 0 to 65 percent.[9] In a 1985 study highly publicized upon its release, Hunter Hansfield, Director of Public Health in Seattle, reported that 5.5 percent of prostitutes were seropositive. As a sample for his study, 92 women in jail for prostitution were forced to give blood for the ELISA test. Not only was his sample unrepresentative of the prostitute population, but his HIV test also generated false positive results. A subsequent, more accurate Western Blot test revealed that none of the women in his sample was seropositive. Hansfield has done nothing to quell the "prostitute panic" his study erroneously fueled. He has yet to publish the updated test results.[10]

In a study conducted shortly after Hansfield's, Project AWARE found that 9 of 146 San Francisco Bay area prostitutes tested HIV positive (6.2 percent). All of them had a history of IV drug use. AWARE found that a sample of sexually active nonprostitute women had similar infection rates, correlating more closely with needle-sharing habits and unprotected sex with needle-sharing men than with prostitution. This study and six others by various groups in this area concluded that the prevalence of seropositivity in prostitutes paralleled the cumulative incidence of AIDS in nonprostitute women. In other words, women who are paid for sex do not contract HIV any more than women who are not.[11]

Unlike prostitutes, johns have not been studied as agents of HIV transmission to sex workers, even though many johns are as sexually active as many sex workers. Only one small unpublished study conducted by Joyce Wallace has attempted to assess the rates at which johns in the United States actually contract HIV. In her sample of 500 johns, only three tested seropositive, claiming no risk behaviors other than sex with women.[12] Evidence indicates that at this time in the

United States, heterosexual men (as a group) engaging in sex with prostitutes (as a group) have not been contracting HIV from them. Female prostitutes, on the other hand, are more likely to contract HIV from unprotected vaginal, anal, or oral sex with men.

All scientific studies must be interpreted in a political context. When reading a study, think about its motives. Think about how the study's recruitment methods affect the results. For example, many early studies recruited subjects from prisons and drug treatment programs, where needle sharing was a likely mode of transmission. Consider the kind of HIV testing done. Was it reliable? Were the results confirmed? Remember that for most men, the least stigmatized mode of HIV transmission is sex with a woman. Men may claim HIV transmission from contact with a prostitute rather than admit to having had sex with another man or to IV drug use.

At this point, it is clear that exposure to body fluids through needle sharing and unprotected sex are the main risk factors for HIV transmission, no matter who you are. Monitoring seroprevalence rates among sex workers for further transmission research is a waste of time and money, especially without substantial improvements in counseling, drug treatment, and health care services for those who need them most.

Discrimination against Prostitutes

> I put prostitutes and gays at about the same level...and I'd be hard-put to give somebody life for killing a prostitute.
>
> Judge Hampton, a Texas judge explaining why he gave a light sentence to men convicted of killing a gay man.[13]

There is a thriving tradition of violence and discrimination against prostitutes. This violence can manifest itself on the street in beatings, rapes, and vigilante attacks on working women. Because prostitution is defined as a crime, sex workers are extended minimal protection under the law. Prostitutes are subject to arrest, quarantine, and mandatory testing for sexually transmitted diseases. Because prostitution is illegal, employers are not responsible to sex workers in any way. Sex workers have no job-related health or disability benefits, making health care difficult to obtain. Economic conditions dictate that seropositive women sometimes have to continue to work during illness. Then, even if safe sex is practiced with clients, sex workers are open to further legal prosecution. In its most benign forms, discrimination against prostitutes is merely insulting. But when police turn a blind eye to crimes committed against sex workers, or when medical scientists only research prostitute seropositivity without providing their subjects treatment and education, it can be deadly.

During World War I, the government quarantined over 30,000 women in response to soaring numbers of syphilis cases, rather than distribute condoms to America's roving servicemen.[14] Any woman under suspicion was forced to test for VD, with devastating personal consequences. Syphilis rates contined to soar. Though never an effective public health measure, quarantine (imprisonment) is now applied in some states to HIV-positive individuals. State quarantine laws not specifically mentioning prostitutes are nonetheless selectively applied to prostitutes. A current South Carolina AIDS law was used to prosecute a Black, mentally disabled prostitute who was placed under house arrest (quarantine) for 90 days because she was HIV positive. Under a similar law in Orlando, Florida, a sex worker was charged with manslaughter, even though she used condoms with all her customers and all her customers tested were seronegative. Seropositive prostitutes are treated extremely harshly, as if they deserve to get AIDS and are hellbent on infecting others. Just imagine the impossibility of a prostitute charging a john with infecting her! In the Nevada counties where registered prostitution is legal, women, not johns, are required to use condoms during sex. Since men are the ones with the penises, wouldn't it make better sense to require johns to make sure condoms are worn during sex?

In 1986, the Food and Drug Administration issued guidelines to blood banks recommending that anyone who has "had sex for money or drugs since 1977" be barred from giving blood. This recommendation stands along with other heterosexist, racist, and faulty prohibitions excluding "any man who has had sexual contact with another man since 1977, even once," and "anyone who was born in or emigrated from Haiti or Africa," except nine exempted countries.[15] Nonprostitutes who have had sex with prostitutes are prohibited from giving blood for only six months, just long enough for HIV antibodies to show up in a routine ELISA test. COYOTE has protested these FDA recommendations, saying the guidelines should advise donors according to risk behavior, not reputation.

Imperialism, Tourism, and the Sex Trade

Many issues for prostitutes around the world stem from policies and attitudes prevailing in this country. As a major world power, the United States sets policy precedents for other countries to follow. Governments dependent on the United States for financial or military support are directly affected by U.S. AIDS policy.

Prostitution is a large component of the Philippine economy. There are over 150,000 Filipinas servicing the tourist industry and the U.S. military. In Manila, over 5 percent of the female population are employed as prostitutes,[16] reflecting the poor economic situation many Filipinas face and the large market there for sex services.

The Subic Naval Base is the largest U.S. naval base off American soil. In Olongapo City, a city of 200,000 people that has sprung up around the base, there are over 10,000 registered "hospitality girls" and countless unregistered street workers.[17] Although prostitution is officially illegal, Philippine law requires that "bar girls" test regularly for HIV and other STDs. Only a portion routinely comply. The U.S. Navy subsidizes the mandatory HIV testing of these women, but does not finance any of the treatments for those who are sick or infected with HIV. The results of VD tests are publicized at the base on a board displaying photographs of the women employed at different night-clubs. U.S. military personnel, of course, are not required to test routinely for STDs for the benefit of Filipina sex workers.

Medical authorities inform women if HIV tests are positive, but neither the ramifications of infection nor the long-term prognosis is discussed. Most women must continue to work. Three months later, seropositive women are taken to the U.S. Naval Hospital in Manila and tested again. There they are given some information about HIV and transmission, but they receive no counseling and no treatment. One Navy doctor involved in AIDS research, Lieutenant Commander Thomas O'Rourke, has indicated that U.S. servicemen are infecting Filipina sex workers with HIV. O'Rourke has since been court-martialed for illegally distributing painkillers to AIDS patients.

The military fails to give adequate education to enlisted troops and the working women servicing them. As a result, many servicemen refuse to use condoms. Filipina bar girls are under great pressure to do what a customer wants, because a dissatisfied customer can get a refund from the bar, usually at her expense. U.S. military men are eager to have sex, but they shirk their responsibility to behave safely with sex partners.

Conclusion

Sex workers are at risk for HIV infection. Clients demanding skin-to-skin contact, lovers expecting the same, arresting officers confiscating condoms, waiting lists for drug treatment programs, and the lack of public health care and drug treatment all jeopardize the health and safety of women sex workers. Legal violence from the state threatens every aspect of a prostitute's existence. Legal, social, and economic obstacles faced by all women become larger when applied to women who sell sex for a living. What's an AIDS activist to do? Support prostitutes' rights organizations. Find out the laws and policies in your area concerning mandatory testing, quarantine, and condom confiscation. And make these demands:

- Decriminalize prostitution.
- Stop scapegoating sex workers for HIV transmission.
- Stop police confiscation of condoms and bleach.
- Educate—let prostitutes teach prostitutes.
- Educate—make johns take responsibility for safe sex.
- Make drug treatment available on demand.
- Make latex barriers free and accessible.

Acknowledgments

Thanks to Priscilla Alexander, CAL-PEP, Tracy Quan, and P.O.N.Y.

Notes

1. Priscilla Alexander, *Prostitutes Prevent AIDS: A Manual for Health Educators* (San Francisco: California Prostitutes Education Project, 1988), p. 56. Available from CAL-PEP, PO Box 6297, San Francisco, CA 94101-6297, (415) 558-0450.
2. "The Highest Paying Customers: America's Cities and the Costs of Prostitution Control," *Hastings Law Journal,* Vol. 38, no. 4, April 1987, pp. 769-800.
3. Frederique Delacoste and Priscilla Alexander, eds., *Sex Work: Writings by Women in the Sex Industry* (Pittsburgh, PA: Cleis Press, 1987), p. 189.
4. Delacoste and Alexander, *Sex Work,* pp. 196-197.
5. Constance Wofsy, "AIDS in Prostitutes: Epidemiology," AIDS Knowledge Base from San Francisco General Hospital (available online from BRS Information Technologies), Waltham, MA: Massachusetts Medical Society, 1988.
6. Delacoste and Alexander, *Sex Work,* p. 248.
7. Alexander, *Prostitutes Prevent* AIDS, p. 3.
8. Alexander, *Prostitutes Prevent AIDS,* p. 39.
9. Michael J. Rosenburg, M.D., M.P.H., and Jodie M. Weiner, M.S.N., "Prostitutes and AIDS: A Health Department Priority?" *American Journal of Public Health,* Vol. 78, no. 4, 1988, pp. 418-423.
10. Alexander, *Prostitutes Prevent AIDS,* p. 33.
11. Alexander, *Prostitutes Prevent AIDS,* p. 33.
12. Joyce Wallace, personal communication, July 1989. Also in "AIDS in Prostitutes," in Pearl Ma and Donald Armstrong, eds., *AIDS and Infections of Homosexual Men* (Boston: Butterworths, 1989). Also updated by Joyce Wallace on *Geraldo,* May 11, 1990.

13. Steven R. Reed, "Judge's 'Queers' Remarks Defended," *Houston Chronicle*, November 14, 1989, p. 27A.
14. Allan M. Brandt, "The Syphilis Epidemic and Its Relation to AIDS," *Science*, Vol. 239, January 1988, p. 377.
15. "What You Need to Know Before You Give Blood," New York Blood Center flyer, March 1990.
16. Freda Guttman, Robert Majzels, and Colette St.-Hilaire, "Daughters of the Dispossessed: Prostitution in the Philippines," *Healthsharing*, Summer 1988, p. 24.
17. Saundra Sturdevant, "The Bar Girls of Subic Bay," *The Nation*, April 3, 1989, p. 444.

Heterosexual Women and AIDS

MONICA PEARL

Although both men and women are at risk for receiving HIV infection from engaging in unprotected sex with each other, women may in fact be at higher risk, just as they have always been at greater risk for contracting sexually transmitted diseases such as chlamydia and gonorrhea. Sex has always been risky for women, and the appearance of HIV provides no exception.

In the United States it is clear that heterosexual women constitute the population that will next be most severely affected by AIDS, even though the mainstream media obscure the real danger with misleading statistics. Considering that the first wave of women now being infected is predominantly women of color, there is a vague and unrealistic sense among most of the straight white female population that AIDS is not their concern. *The New York Times,* in a dubious attempt, perhaps, to reassure the defensively named "general population" that there is little for those outside certain so-called "risk groups" to fear, asserts in an article entitled "Spread of AIDS By Heterosexuals Remains Slow"[1] that "only about 5 percent of the full-fledged AIDS cases in this country have been officially attributed to heterosexual transmission." Only when you reach the follow-up page and scrutinize the accompanying graph do you realize that this 5 percent breaks down into 2 percent of all cases in men and *31 percent in women.* Slow for whom, one might ask. Twenty-four paragraphs into the article we find that "cases attributed to heterosexual transmission are growing faster than any other category of AIDS cases."

When the media refer to heterosexual AIDS as a myth, they seem to suggest that "heterosexual" must not include women, because AIDS for heterosexual women is not only not a myth, but is what, in some cities, is most likely to kill them. In New York City, for example,

AIDS is the leading cause of death for women aged 25 to 34, taking nearly three times as many lives as the second and third leading causes of death for women in this age group, drug dependence and cancer.[2] Not only does heterosexual seem to mean only men, but it seems to mean only white, as it is women of color who constitute the population of heterosexual women who are currently most severely affected by the AIDS crisis. Referring to heterosexual AIDS as a myth is genocidal. Privilege won't protect you from HIV, and neither will lies.

Some of the most egregious misinformation concerning heterosexual women and AIDS appears in *The Real Truth About Women and AIDS* by Helen Singer Kaplan.[3] Kaplan unrealistically exhorts women to avoid any sexual activity with any man about whose sexual or drug-using history we are uncertain, claiming that condoms and any form of safe sex aside from abstinence are insufficient. "Clearly," she writes, "the best strategy for you is to avoid sex with high-risk men, and if you are not sure whether a man has or has not been exposed," she blithely continues, "do not go to bed with him until he is tested and cleared." First, there is no such thing as a high-risk individual; there is only high-risk behavior. Second, not only is it unrealistic to expect that women will insist that their potential (or current) sexual partners be tested before having sex, it is unnecessary. For one thing, one negative test does not account for the incubation period of HIV (largely held to be at least six months) that would render a negative test result misleading. The safest and wisest course is to insist on and practice safer sex, whether this includes condoms or finding ways to be sexual without the exchange of blood or semen. "Women," Kaplan proselytizes, "have the power and the obligation to guard the general population from the incoming infestation…Our bodies," she continues, "form a protective ring around the breeding grounds of the AIDS virus." Men, in other words, won't do it for themselves or for us, so we must ourselves be the hygienic and moralistic gatekeepers of the world.

So far, the greatest cries of concern regarding heterosexual women and AIDS have been narrowly directed, primarily, at saving the "innocent" potential lives of unborn children, and, ironically, by counseling HIV-positive women toward abortion and sterilization rather than providing medical care and treatment.

Perhaps the most severe and subtle problem around the issue of AIDS prevention for all women having sex with men is precisely how to negotiate safer sex with our lovers. While the negotiation and practice of safer sex should never be, exclusively, the woman's responsibility, it is clear that under most circumstances, as has been the case historically with birth control, if a woman doesn't take care of things for herself, no one else will. The fact is that many straight men find safer sex—specifically, the use of condoms—either hateful or unnecessary and will go to varying lengths, depending on their degree of distaste, to avoid using them. For many women who sleep with men, the fear of becoming infected with HIV is insignificant in comparison to the fear of reprisal involved in even suggesting to their lovers that they use condoms. Anticipated and actual reactions range from ridicule to physical violence. Many women are choosing to stop having sex or to continue to have unsafe sex rather than taking on what seems like the insurmountable task of negotiating safer sex.

One of the most prevalent conditions of transmission of HIV is the regular practice of unsafe sex among those who continue to believe that they are not at risk, who cannot convince their partners to practice safer sex, or who are lied to about the degree of knowledge their partners have about their HIV status. That is to say, some women who believe that their sexual partner or partners present them with no risk are wrong. If your lover, for example, tells you that he has tested negative and that he won't have sex with anyone else but you, you have to agree to believe and trust him or else you have to practice safe sex. He has only to have sex with someone else once to put you in danger. Also, just as birth control created some sexual flexibility for women, so does practicing safe sex, even with your primary partner, because then you can constantly make choices about when and with whom to be sexual without putting yourself or your partner at risk. Another option is to agree to practice safer-sex with all partners but your primary partner, but again, this requires that you are both HIV-negative and can trust each other to be thorough and practical *always*. Safe sex is for everyone—not only for those who suspect they might be at risk.

The incorporation of safer-sex techniques into a sexual relationship can actually be liberating for women in moving the focus of sex away from penis and vagina and away from the idea that sex must be always and only intercourse. In fact, for women who have always felt that they were not made love to properly by men, who weren't touched or aroused in the way they wanted, the introduction of safer sex into a relationship can be nearly revolutionary. Rather than merely introducing barriers or inconveniences, safer sex has the profound potential to eroticize sex. It can be an opportunity to experiment with nonpenetrative ways of turning each other on.

Safe sex, practiced consistently and correctly, not only protects both partners from HIV, but also provides effective birth control, and effectively protects women and men from just about all sexually transmitted diseases. So, although there seem to be many prospective dangers against which women have to protect themselves during sex, safe sex satisfies all these protective criteria. If you know you are HIV positive, practicing safe sex allows you to continue being sexual without risking transmission to your partner, and also protects your own health, as repeated contact with the virus can accelerate the infection. It's *your* body and *your* life; you can protect yourself and have great sex.

The only way we're going to get through the AIDS crisis is by taking care of ourselves and each other. This means not only educating ourselves but agitating for information and consideration. Organize teach-ins around the issues of safer sex; don't let anyone tell you to stop being sexual or to have sex that isn't safe. It has been for too long that women have been told how and when to have sex. So have sex—and do it safely.

Notes

1. Philip J. Hilts, "Spread of AIDS by Heterosexuals Remains Slow," *The New York Times,* May 1, 1990, pp. C1 and C12.
2. Bruce Lambert, "AIDS Deaths Near Another Awful Record," *The New York Times,* March 25, 1990, p. E20.
3. Helen Singer Kaplan, *The Real Truth About Women and AIDS* (New York: Simon and Schuster, 1987).

Demanding a Condom

KAT DOUD

Before I understood AIDS, who got it, and how it could be prevented, I was scared, really scared. I felt at risk but for the wrong reasons. I was afraid of casual contact with people instead of being afraid of having unsafe sex with a man I was seeing at the time. Max (not his real name) was putting a lot of pressure on me to get birth control pills for protection, only the only protection pills would offer would be for pregnancy—not AIDS. During this time, my fear of AIDS was growing. I was getting really paranoid, so I called the hotline. They talked a lot about condoms and safer sex. I went immediately to Max to tell him how I was feeling and that I wouldn't have sex with him without condoms. His reaction was horrible. He got very angry and full of contempt and accused me of having AIDS, and angry that I insinuated that he did. I began to try to explain, then realized he wasn't worth my time. Why would I want to sleep with this creature who didn't care about my life? I never saw him again after that night.

Bisexual Women and AIDS

ALEXIS DANZIG

AC/DC. AM/FM. The double-gaited set. The nicknames have always been a little nasty. One view commonly held by therapists and gay activists is that bisexuals are merely self-deceived homosexuals, "fence-sitters," unwilling to face up to their same-sex preference. Heterosexuals tend to think of "bi's" as the ultimate libertines, the ones determined to "have it all." As one bisexual once put it, "Why should we be prevented from sleeping with half the human race?" There is now a very short answer to that question, a four-letter word that explains why bisexuals are becoming the ultimate pariahs of the '80s. That word is AIDS.

Newsweek, July 13, 1987

Bisexual women exist. Like lesbians we can be at risk for AIDS through unsafe contact with the blood or vaginal fluids of HIV-positive women; like straight women we can be at risk through unsafe contact with the blood or semen of HIV-positive men. If we shoot drugs we can be at risk from sharing works with others who are HIV positive. And, like all women in the United States, we are at risk for AIDS because women are denied specific, usable information about preventing HIV transmission and because we must look for this life-saving information in an AIDS-phobic and sex-negative social climate.

The AIDS crisis brings up issues for bisexual women that our monosexual sisters may never have to face. AIDS presents us with multiple issues of power and powerlessness that our exclusively lesbian and straight sisters may share with us in part, but that as bisexual women we must learn to confront in our own ways.

Who Defines Bisexuality? What Is "Being Bisexual"?

Bisexuals, unlike most self-conscious gay/lesbian people and the overwhelming majority of straight people, have few or no outlets for self-expression and understanding other than through our personal sexual relationships. While mainstream culture is dominantly heterosexual, strong gay and lesbian subcultures exist around the world, and in most Western cities gay and lesbian publications, bars, and organizations can be found. Bisexual people have few places where we can go to "be bisexual"; few publications exist for us to communicate and discuss among ourselves what "being bisexual" means to us. Finally, because we so often lack written histories and traditions, we cannot develop widespread consciousness of ourselves or political agendas for ourselves. As a result, many of us who behave bisexually—who enjoy sex with both men and women—in fact identify as either gay or straight.

But whether we are the publicly or self-identified bisexual woman who relates sexually to men and women, the straight woman who has slept with her female roommate for the first time, or the lesbian who occasionally fucks her best gay male buddy, we are often misrepresented and typically misunderstood by others. Both straight and gay people seem more concerned with speaking for us than hearing from us.

According to the *Newsweek* article quoted, "therapists" (unspecified but presumably straight) and "gay activists" perceive bisexuals as existing in a state of denial, "unwilling to face up to their same-sex preference." But it is the straights in this article who deny all *connection* between themselves and bisexuals, while the gay people deny any *difference* between themselves and bisexuals.

Both groups' denial masks the fact that many people experience their sexual identities apart from their social identities. Both groups' denial tries to hide the issue that sexual behaviors can be and often are more complicated and diverse than the sociosexual definitions "homosexual," "heterosexual," and even "bisexual" will allow.

For many women, the only time we might think about our bisexuality is when we are experiencing a contradiction between how we identify ourselves publicly, and what we feel and do, emotionally and sexually, in private. We might be beginning a new relationship with someone we're not "supposed" to fall in love with, or thinking about our attraction to a person with the "wrong" body, or wondering what it means that we made love with someone unexpected last night. Experiencing a difference between our gay or straight public identity and the private experience of our sexuality can be scary and threatening, at the same time that we feel turned on and powerful about this aspect and this expression of our sexuality.

Privately I know I'm bisexual—I'm sexual with men and women. But the term "bisexual" is so empty. Bisexual people aren't "serious." I define myself as a lesbian, but if I'm feeling really brave I'll say I'm a lesbian-identified bisexual.

Three years ago I was definitely a lesbian. Now I think of myself as bisexual, sometimes. One thing I'm sure of is latex. Oh, and nonoxynol-9 lube.

Some of us may identify publicly as bisexuals and may not feel this conflict within ourselves; yet outwardly we too may feel the need to choose between groups with whom we socialize and do political work. We may experience that it is "easier" for us to be with a certain group at a certain time or because of a particular issue. If we publicly identify as bisexuals we may feel pressure from lesbians and straight women to "make a real commitment" or "stop being confused." We may experience pressure to hide aspects of ourselves that might threaten monosexual people. Or we might choose to be silent about these parts of ourselves because: (a) it's our business, we're comfortable with it and don't need to share it; (b) we don't want to upset those around us; (c) we don't want to make ourselves vulnerable to others' judgments and speculations, or risk rejection.

I wanted her so much that I couldn't bring myself to tell her that I'd just gotten out of a relationship with a guy. He and I had always used rubbers so I wasn't worried about AIDS. I was just worried about losing her. When I told her, one evening when we'd just made love, I was feeling very bold and very vulnerable. She said, "Life's complicated," and held me in her arms.

Bisexuality and Heterosexism

Heterosexism is the assumption—accepted by individuals and perpetuated by and enforced through institutions—that heterosexuality is superior to other sexualities and is the only natural kind of sexuality. Heterosexism affects bisexual people in several ways. First, heterosexism accounts for most of the hostility bisexual people experience. It is our *same*-sex relationships or relationship potential that challenge the heterosexual norm. As bisexual women, we may find that we are pressured not to discuss our female lovers with straight friends and relatives, while our relationships with men are celebrated.

I'd been out as a lesbian for three years when I came out to my kid brother. At the time I had a bed-buddy who was male. My brother's comment to me when I told him "I'm a lesbian" was, "Yeah, right."

Because of our lesbian relationships we may be discriminated against as lesbians have been and are: at work and at school, in housing and in health care. We may find that our lesbianism is dismissed by social workers and psychiatrists who expect us to "outgrow" our "immature" love of women. Or, conversely, as implied in the *Newsweek* article, therapists may negate us as self-deluded in our dual sexual identification, dismissing us *as* lesbians.

Heterosexism also helps set the tone for the way bisexuals are received in gay and lesbian circles. Many bisexual people feel comfortable socially, politically, and sexually with gay men and lesbians. But for some gay and lesbian people who have been intolerantly treated by straight society, we may be viewed as cowardly, as sexual tourists, and even as traitors with access to heterosexual privileges gay men and lesbians can never or would never seek to enjoy. For gay and lesbian people, straight privilege might be something desired, like having access to health care merely because of a publicly sanctioned relationship; or it might be something seen as undesirable to most gay and lesbian people, but something that is nonetheless status conferring, like being accepted as straight.

While many bisexual women do not have full straight privileges and may only be perceived as straight by those who don't know us (a common presumption in a predominantly heterosexual culture), we may be resented for appearing to have more choices open to us, including the "choice" not to "be" lesbians. But those of us who identify as lesbians often do not feel that we are *choosing not* to be lesbians; rather, it is our *choice,* as lesbians, to be sexual with a man or men. As lesbians who sleep with men, if we are public with our experience, we may be condemned by lesbians who claim that "real lesbians don't sleep with men."

> I picked up the phone and my boyfriend's ex-boyfriend was screaming at me, "You're a lesbian, you're supposed to fuck girls!" And I thought, "He should tell that to my mother." I'm being flip about it now but at the time it was really painful, like I was being rejected by my own community.

Bisexuals and AIDS

In the current hysteria of AIDS-phobia, bisexual women are overlooked and ignored by medical authorities and the government agencies designed to facilitate health care, while being vilified as "vectors" of HIV transmission to lesbians—a population whose needs for AIDS information and awareness are also generally trivialized or forgotten.

> I remember finding out that my friend's girlfriend is HIV positive.

It completely changed their lives. It wasn't a matter for them to choose to have safer sex or not. If they wanted to make love it had to be safer sex. For the rest of their lives. Now it bugs me when I hear other lesbians talk about bisexuals and how they give lesbians AIDS. This woman had been an IVDU—she did needle drugs before, but she'd been clean for about seven years. But lesbians don't face the fact that lesbians can get AIDS from shooting drugs. We don't talk about addiction and how to clean needles, but we'll get pissed off at the *idea* of bisexual women. I think that sucks.

That women who are sexual with both men and women are important, worth keeping informed, healthy, and alive is lost in discussions of epidemiology ("can women transmit HIV to men?") and in statements of blame ("bisexual women spread HIV to lesbians"). Here heterosexism becomes deadly to bisexual women. Safer-sex and drug-use education rarely address those of us who are bisexually active.

Our understanding of HIV transmission can be as piecemeal and as faulty as the way it was presented to us. For instance, we may have a clear understanding of using condoms for sex with men, but may never have heard of dental dams for sex with women because the organization from which we received our AIDS information failed to fully address lesbian sexuality and HIV prevention. And finally, because of the general anxiety about and anger at bisexual people from both straight and gay people, we may find it overwhelmingly difficult to be open about and to negotiate safer sex and drug use with our partners.

People, even people I've known for a while who know that I sleep with women and men, will ask me why I continue to sleep with men, some of whom are gay. They say, "Why don't you just sleep with women?"—as if I could just turn off my attraction to men. These people don't know anything about desire—or, perhaps more importantly, about safer sex. On some level they must think that being gay means you must have AIDS and therefore can't have sex anymore. These people scare me more than Jesse Helms. Some of the hottest sex I've had has been safer sex.

Because of heterosexism, bisexual women are at risk for HIV transmission as well as for the increased violence against people perceived as sexually different. It is important that lesbians who sleep with men, straight women who sleep with women, and self-identified bisexual women begin creating awareness of our sexualities, of our experiences with safer sex and HIV transmission, with each other and with our monosexual sisters. Together with informed lesbians and straight women we have the collective potential to challenge dominant misperceptions about all the women in the AIDS crisis, as well as to confront the heterosexist fear of differences that controls so many aspects of our lives and choices. As women who are sexual with both men and women, reclaiming our bisexualities can empower us against disinformation and allow us to redefine for ourselves what "being bisexual" can mean about taking responsibility for ourselves and those we love in the AIDS crisis.

Acknowledgments

Many thanks to my friends, the women and men whose conversations with me over several years have contributed greatly to ideas expressed and voices heard in this essay.

Reproductive Rights and AIDS: The Connections

MARION BANZHAF

TRACY MORGAN

KAREN RAMSPACHER

The Feminist Health Movement: Background for Reproductive Rights

Were it not for the feminist health movement of the 1970s, there would be no "Know Your Body" classes, no Patient's Bill of Rights, no birthing centers in hospitals, fewer women doctors, and no view that "patients" are also consumers. The feminist health movement not only redefined women's health *as* health and not disease, and provided institutional alternatives for health care, but also confronted the medical establishment as an industry that was sexist, racist, and classist in its treatment of women. The successes and failures of that movement provide valuable lessons for the AIDS movement.

The politics of the feminist health movement were radical and far reaching. Five basic principles were

- Women's medical treatment was part of women's oppression: as a rule, all women received sexist treatment.
- Women needed to seize control of women's health and demystify common procedures.
- Collectivity, in both the operation and provision of health services, politicized health care and deprivatized women's common experiences, thus extending the tenet "the personal is political" to health.
- The feminist health movement and women's clinics needed to operate autonomously from the state.
- Service work done in a political context was political, and women deserved to be paid for their work.

Women's Medical Treatment as Part of Women's Oppression

The feminist health movement developed from the women's liberation movement of the late 1960s. Using techniques of consciousness-raising (CR), women realized that most of us had experienced humiliating, degrading, and often abusive maltreatment from male doctors. The Boston Women's Health Book Collective developed from a CR group and published *Our Bodies, Ourselves* in 1969. *Our Bodies, Ourselves* was the first information about women's health written by and for women. It galvanized women to start talking and acting—about sex, birth control, abortion, childbirth, and lesbianism. Distributed nationally, it enabled women to learn what our doctors had been doing behind our backs and between our legs.

The operating principle was that women couldn't control our own lives until we could control our bodies. Since women's "health" and "illness" had always been reproductively defined, the medical profession viewed the totality of women's experiences through our uteruses.

The feminist health movement set out to change the definition of women's health from a disease model to a health model. For example, pregnancy is not a disease, and since doctors are schooled in disease, not health, women challenged their relationships to doctors and medical institutions.

Part of this confrontation meant fighting for the principle that every woman could understand her anatomy, could learn basic health maintenance measures, and so informed could make autonomous decisions about her health. Many health projects developed training programs for laywomen to become health workers and educators. Recognizing women's history as healers, the feminist health movement wanted to put women's health back into women's hands and openly opposed the historical hoarding of health information by professionals.

Fighting AIDS

On December 15, 1975, the newly formed National Women's Health Network held its first demonstration—a memorial service in front of the Food and Drug Administration (FDA) in Rockville, Maryland—to commemorate the thousands of women who had died from synthetic-estrogen-related complications. On October 11, 1988, AIDS activists stood on the same ground demanding that the FDA respond to their needs and heed the deaths of tens of thousands from AIDS.

Reproductive rights and AIDS activism are intimately connected. Both movements are committed to claiming political control over the body. Both movements focus on health care and self-empowerment. Both movements address issues at the core of how our society is organized economically and sexually.

The movement for reproductive rights grew, in part, out of the movement for abortion rights. Reproductive rights encompass far more than abortion rights. Not everyone's view of reproductive control focuses on abortion. Reproductive rights include the right to sex without punishment and without unplanned pregnancy, the right to have sex with whom we want, and the right to sex without risk of illness, including HIV infection. They also include the right to determine whether and when we want to have children, the right to have healthy children and accessible child care, and the right to quality health services and control over our health care decisions. The movement for reproductive rights has grown to reflect diverse reproductive issues.

But this broadened view evolved only from directly confronting issues of racism and classism. Linking abortion rights with a struggle against sterilization abuse started in the early 1970s, when Black, Native American, and Puerto Rican women began to expose sterilization abuses in their communities. Sterilization of teenagers, consent obtained during labor, hysterectomies performed for sterilization, sterilization required by a physician as a condition for delivering a baby, and consent forms written in English for non-English-speaking women were some of the abuses that resulted in much higher rates of sterilization among women of color and poor white women than among white middle-class women. The National Abortion Rights Action League, Planned Parenthood, and the National Organization for Women did not support grassroots efforts to stop sterilization abuses by creating federal regulations, including a mandatory 30-day waiting period.

These groups, representing the interests of white middle-class women, considered these regulations an infringement on women's right to choose. The Committee for Abortion Rights and Against Sterilization Abuse (CARASA) and the Committee to End Sterilization Abuse organized to fight abuses that poor women and women of color experienced, linking these issues to all women's right to reproductive freedom. In 1978, federal guidelines incorporating a waiting period and native language consent forms were issued. That struggle incorporated some demands of women of color into what remains a predominantly white middle-class reproductive rights agenda.

Opposing racism and classism is essential in the fight against AIDS. AIDS activism first emerged in the economically advantaged, white, gay male community. For some of these men, the AIDS crisis became their first direct experience of institutionalized oppression. Even while confronted with gay oppression through lack of governmental response to the AIDS crisis, the gay white male community could muster considerable resources. Public and private funding sources have boosted activity in the gay community (e.g., the Gay Men's Health Crisis) while other AIDS political and service groups have had to fend for what's left. Rather than share resources and acknowledge common bonds, the white, gay AIDS activist movement initially embraced a single-issue strategy (getting new drugs into bodies) and didn't consider the needs of women, intravenous drug users (IVDUs), and children. Fortunately, this strategy is changing. Lesbian, bisexual, and straight women, and women and gay men of color joined the gay AIDS activist movement to get our concerns onto the agenda. Autonomous groups have developed to work on issues affecting women, IVDUs, and ethnic communities (e.g., African-American, Haitian, Asian, Native American, Puerto Rican). Increasingly, AIDS activists are striving to build coalitions that will focus on broad survival issues, such as universal health care, decent housing, home health care, child care, treatment for children with AIDS, protection of legal rights, expanded detoxification and drug counseling programs, and prisoners' rights.

The Sex Connection

The fight for reproductive rights is, among other things, a fight for sexual pleasure. We live in a world where many women feel awkward referring explicitly to parts of our bodies. Many of us do not masturbate, or don't admit it. Even talking about birth control and safer sex with our partners can be hard. These examples demonstrate how women, as a group, have been denied access to our physical selves. Without control over our bodies, we have little control over our lives.

Attacking reproductive control by limiting abortion rights limits the independence of all women and, by extension, polices female desire. Eroticism, from a reproductive rights perspective, is power—a power that, up until 20 years ago, had been kept far from the reaches of many women. As Audre Lorde writes, "In touch with the erotic, I become less willing to accept powerlessness."[1] When we take back our bodies as sites of pleasure for ourselves, we challenge the whole structure of power in our culture that dictates who can ask for pleasure and who must service others' desires.

AIDS activists are also involved in the fight for sexual pleasure.

Many public policymakers, politicians, religious leaders, and others have exploited this health crisis by encouraging people to be sexually abstinent until marriage. Aside from the blatant heterosexism of this kind of thinking, urging abstinence plays into the U.S. public's pleasure/guilt complex and basic fear of sex. Given the sensationalist media coverage of AIDS, it is not surprising that the pressure is on for people (especially women) to avoid the bedroom. But the answer to AIDS prevention does not lie in abstinence. It lies in safer-sex education and practice.

To have safe sex we have to talk about sex, what it means to us, and how we do it. Eroticism, from an AIDS activist perspective, requires protection both in the form of latex and in a militant pro-sex attitude. Again, Audre Lorde's words do great justice:

> When we begin to live from within outward, in touch with the power of the erotic within ourselves, and allowing that power to inform and illuminate our actions upon the world around us, then we begin to be responsible to ourselves in the deepest sense.[2]

The gay community was not about to give up the thriving, homoerotic culture it had worked so hard to create. In the 1970s, gay men came out of the closet and actually had somewhere to go. Bar culture was exciting. Bathhouses thrived. Gay businesses flourished. But the inroads toward claiming gay identity had been made for gay men—by gay men. No one from outside the community had done it any great favors. So, when AIDS was called "the gay cancer," and public health officials stormed bathhouses to close them down, the gay male community was still on its own.

The reproductive rights movement has a parallel history. Thanks to 1970s feminism, women deprivatized sex and were encouraged to cultivate our clitoral orgasmic pleasures. Vaginal orgasm was debunked as a myth. The move to affirm female sexuality gave visibility to lesbian and bisexual women. We could and would have sex with whom we wanted. The "pill" removed the awkwardness from birth control, and abortion was legalized. We had our own desires and could act on them as we saw fit (until the 1977 passage of the Hyde Amendment wiped out federal Medicaid funds for abortions). But today we find that many women's health facilities have gone out of business. The elimination of Title X funds to family planning clinics that only provide counseling about abortion has closed smaller clinics. Or, we arrive at a facility and find Operation Rescue blockading the entrance, protected by the police.

Both movements have been hounded by the moral specter of

sex guilt. In the early-to-mid-1980s, the media declared that gay men had "done themselves in" by having "too much sex." The attitude of many public figures is that homosex is unnatural and AIDS is a deserved punishment. This conservatism was expressed in an editorial in an American gay sex magazine that moralized: "It's time to be discreet…just quit being such a flighty dick-pig, bath house queen, indiscreet butt-chaser and uncontrollable whore."[3]

Feminists also accepted certain antiabortion rhetoric. Betty Friedan, at the 1989 National Abortion Rights Action League conference, implied in her speech that abortion is a necessary evil. The time when women did not have to apologize or feel guilty seemed long gone. But heightened activism following the Supreme Court's 1989 *Webster* decision is challenging once again the terms of the abortion debate. By calling abortion "murder," those who oppose abortion rights give heterosex an extra-moral aspect for women. Even though a man and a woman engage in sex together, only the woman is blamed for ending an unwanted pregnancy. As antiabortionist Elwood Rudd says, "If a woman has a right to control her own body, let her exercise her control before she gets pregnant."[4] Our control is usurped by a conservative agenda enacted by lawmakers and abortion foes, equating abortion with murder and women with incubators.

AIDS and reproductive rights activists have accelerated their pro-sex politics. In actuality, we cannot teach people about sexuality without including a discussion of dental dams, condoms, nonoxynol-9, birth control, abortion, pregnancy, and orgasm. Birth control research is part of the reproductive rights agenda. Safer sex is also birth control. Feminists have been handing out condoms on street corners for years. We know also, as "Jane Post-Webster" wrote in *Outweek* magazine, "Sex has never been safe for women because of the threat of unwanted pregnancy, rape, and sexual harassment. Women have a stake in fighting for sex to be safe."[5]

The abortion connection to safer-sex education and empowerment of people with AIDS has been hard for some people to grasp. AIDS activists have learned that the health care system in this country is an atrocity. It is discriminatory to the core and continues to give people different care depending on their economic status, race, sex, sexuality, and physical ability. Patient power has grown from these realizations. People with AIDS must become experts about their bodies, HIV treatments, and wellness maintenance. This mode of empowerment through knowledge harks back to the women's self-help health movement of the 1970s. Having an abortion is a decision women make to control our bodies and, in so doing, control our destinies. No one can make the decision for us. And, what we hope will become an integral part of reproductive rights rhetoric is the slogan "Abortion is Health Care." At this point its legitimacy as health care is not recognized. Women are hard pressed to find insurance policies that cover abortion, at the same time that people with AIDS find their insurance terminated upon diagnosis.

The sexist double standard of sexuality is translated by both reproductive rights activists and AIDS activists into a common struggle for control over our bodies and our lives. ACT UP New York and the New York-based Women's Health Action Mobilization (WHAM!) planned a "Stop the Church" demonstration at St. Patrick's Cathedral in New York City on December 10, 1989, with joint demands against the church's opposition to abortion and its murderous AIDS policy.

Broadening our View

Pronatalist (probirth) attitudes, combined with a conservative economic and political base, promote motherhood as an "experience not to be missed" and as women's duty. Hence the contemporary emphasis in popular culture on the ticking of women's biological clocks. Motherhood has always been a biological option for women, and can be quite rewarding, but let's not romanticize it. Motherhood remains primarily a woman's burden, with very few support systems in place. It alters our lives dramatically while men still don't share responsibility equally.

Children are valued differently in different cultures. Most women experience pressure and/or responsibility to have children. A woman might experience a particular desire to have children if genocide is part of her history. A gay white man might have difficulty understanding why a Puerto Rican woman with AIDS wants to have a baby, but since 33 percent of Puerto Rican women have been sterilized, she may see having a child as one way of resisting the genocide of her people.

There has always been discrimination against gay men. But with AIDS, heterosexism becomes both more intense and more obvious. Some gay men have recognized that the system won't take care of them. Funding for AIDS research continues to come slowly and reluctantly from the U.S. government. Clearly, were AIDS a disease initially believed to strike white, heterosexual, upper-class men, funding for research and treatment would have been plentiful. AIDS politicized gay men in the 1980s just as sterilization abuse, valium addiction, dangerous IUDs, DES, and the illegality of abortion politicized women in the 1960s and 1970s.

As the issues overlap, so do the obstacles that prevent women and PWAs from having their full rights under the law. Population policies have always influenced, though sometimes in hidden ways, women's reproductive decisions. In the 1930s, eugenicists advocated sterilizing "undesirables," by whom they meant anyone with disabilities, poor people, and people of color. At the same time, Nazis were coming into power in Germany and planning the extermination of Jews, gays, communists, and others. Now, people with HIV may become the next targets of both passive and aggressive genocidal policies, through mandatory testing, negligent health care, coerced abortions, and calls for quarantine.

Economic policies dictate that "choice" becomes an option only for those with money. Many people who use clinics as their primary source of health care can't afford private physicians and hospitals. The cost of AZT for a year ($8,000) is as much or more than the annual income of some women with AIDS. Poor women and women of color are disproportionately affected by the political and cultural conservatism that reigns in the United States. Women with money can get quality child care and health services no matter what the political climate.

A political view that fights access to health care based on ability to pay and that supports individual decision making will achieve deeper results than a single-issue politic of "drugs into bodies." The union of reproductive rights issues with AIDS activism forces a deeper examination of how to get what we need without violating each other's rights.

Reproductive Issues Affecting HIV-Positive Women

HIV-positive women confront the denial of reproductive control on a number of fronts: they are denied access to experimental treatments based on their reproductive potential, counseled to abort pregnancies they might want to complete, denied abortions by fearful practitioners, and subjected to societal judgments about all their decisions. AIDS research about reproductive issues has been low priority.

No one knows the effect of experimental treatments on women's reproductive organs. AZT was approved without having been tested on women and before animal testing had been concluded. In 1989, Burroughs-Wellcome, the manufacturer of the drug, announced that AZT caused cancer in the reproductive organs of female rats and mice. The AIDS activist agenda has always pushed for accelerated drug approval, but this may represent a conflict between the interests of men and women in the AIDS epidemic, since drugs affect men and women differently. If the specific opportunistic infections of HIV disease in women had been dealt with earlier in the crisis, research on safety and efficacy in women's bodies would not be lagging so far behind.

Profit, not safety, is the primary motivation of pharmaceutical companies. For two generations, women have been experiencing toxic effects of "new" drugs such as thalidomide and DES, and devices such as the copper 7 and Dalkon shield IUDs. The birth control pill was marketed in the United States in the 1960s after a trial of 132 Puerto Rican women in which 2 women died and were then "excluded" from the study report.[6]

The experimental use of DES to prevent miscarriage in approximately 3 million pregnant women between 1945 and 1970 resulted in cancer and death for thousands of their daughters, and testicular cancer in their sons (although in smaller numbers). It took nearly as long to establish that the drug didn't work as to reveal how dangerous it was.

Drug companies' and medical institutions' concern about financial liability for potential fetal damage has kept women out of many drug trials. Certainly many drugs might cause damage to a woman or a fetus, but a woman facing HIV disease may be willing to take the risk. Drug companies and doctors should not be allowed to withhold treatments by pitting a potential fetus against the health of the woman. At the same time, we cannot fall into the trap of prioritizing a PWA's need for drug access over a pregnant woman's concern for that drug's potential damage to her fetus. As with all political conflicts that have bearing on women's lives, it must be our priority to establish policies of full access, informed consent, and the right of an individual to make her own decision, while continuing to press for research on all fronts.

Women and men have different reproductive organs, but our biological differences must not be used against us. Research must be conducted to gain information necessary for women to make informed decisions. In order for information to be available, we demand faster trials on the reproductive organs of female animals. Only from those results will women be able to determine in any truly informed way what risks they are willing to take.

One of the primary reproductive rights issues for HIV-positive women is support for their right to have children if they so desire. The current emphasis on testing women for HIV early in pregnancy is geared more toward preventing the birth of a potentially HIV-infected baby than on providing the woman with better health care. Although the HIV-antibody test only shows *her* status, she is often faced with policies of directed counseling, suggesting abortion. Yet research indicates that the risk of an HIV-positive woman's having an HIV-infected baby is only 20 to 50 percent. Similarly, women need to know that pregnancy does not seem to accelerate HIV disease if the woman is asymptomatic. In other words, having a baby won't make her sicker. If an HIV-positive woman wants to have a baby, the best time for her own health (and potentially the health of the baby) is while she is asymptomatic.

If an HIV-positive woman gets pregnant and doesn't want to continue the pregnancy, she may experience discrimination. A survey of New York City abortion clinics revealed that 64 percent of them denied HIV-positive women an appointment for an abortion.[7] Additionally, HIV-positive women have a hard time finding gynecological care that addresses their particular needs.

Abortion rights activists are considering underground distribution of the new abortion pill, RU486, currently available only in France, using PWA Buyers Clubs as a model. However, many questions about RU486 must be raised, particularly the effects on women with chronic health problems, poor nutrition, or other factors not included in the French studies of middle-class women. Much more research must be done before we will know the effects of RU486 on women with HIV illnesses.

Further, there are some experimental AIDS drugs that are now used in trials that are known to have specific effects on women's bodies. Compound Q, used in China as an abortifacient, certainly will have a specific effect on women's reproductive organs. Megace, a synthetic progestin (female hormone), is being used currently in trials for AIDS patients with wasting syndrome, or severe weight loss. This hormone will have different effects on women's bodies.

These are not easy questions with easy answers. Women's issues must become part of all activists' demands where treatment and drugs are concerned. Improved data will emerge only when we fight for it.

We need to speed up animal reproductive organ testing. Women should not be excluded from trials, but need additional informed consent protection. Women must create the demands that become part of the activist agenda.

Acknowledgments

Risa Denenberg also contributed to this essay.

Notes

1. Audre Lorde, "Uses of the Erotic," *Sister Outsider* (Trumansburg, NY: The Crossing Press Feminist Series, 1984), p. 58.
2. Lorde, "Uses of the Erotic."
3. Simon Watney, *Policing Desire: Pornography, AIDS and the Media* (Minneapolis: University of Minnesota Press, 1989), 2nd ed., p. 19.
4. Ann Snitow, Christine Stansell, and Sharon Thompson, eds., *Powers of Desire: The Politics of Sexuality* (New York: Monthly Review Press, 1983), p. 474.
5. Jane Post-Webster, "Sisters Doing it for Themselves," *Outweek*, September 24, 1989, p. 28.
6. Sheryl Burt Ruzek, *The Women's Health Movement: Feminist Alternatives to Medical Control* (New York: Praeger Publishers, 1978), p. 37.
7. Katherine Franke, Abstract, *V International Conference on AIDS* (June 4-6, 1989), p. 855.

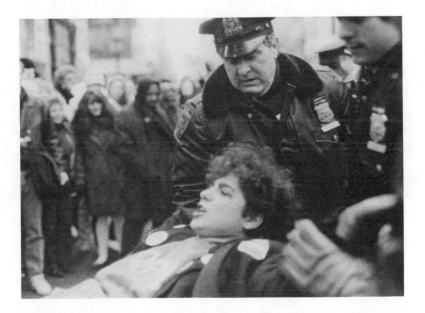

ACT UP and Women's Health Action Mobilization "Stop the Church" at St. Patrick's Cathedral, New York City, December 10, 1989, to protest Cardinal O'Connor's opposition to safe-sex education, abortion rights, and antidiscrimination legislation to protect lesbians and gay men.

Photo by Zoe Leonard

Translating Issues into Actions: Introduction

RACHEL LURIE

Just as we were putting the finishing touches on this book, I got word that a friend of mine from ACT UP had died of AIDS. I wanted to put the book aside that day, to let the news set in slowly, to sit and mourn. How do I reconcile my grief with an impending deadline? More importantly, since this whole project is about AIDS activism, what is the place for my sadness in my militancy? I realized that the loss that makes me sad is the same loss that makes me angry, and it is both of those that propel my activism. One does not replace the other. In part, it is the senseless dying and suffering that propel me to do this work, and it is a suffering that I am not separate from. I want to create a sane world amid the chaos that has begun to take it over. With others, I can be powerful in the face of a disease, a health care system, and a social fabric that threaten to make us all feel powerless. I want to be strengthened in direct proportion to all the beatings that are bestowed upon me. I will fight back for all of us, including those who can fight no more. I reject the analysis that I might be doing AIDS activism out of some altruistic or maternal sense. I am fighting for my own life.

The information throughout this book is critical for us as activists. The very fact that it takes a fight to get this information, that it is not readily available and aggressively reported to the public, is cause enough for our activism. And then the knowledge itself motivates us further, empowering us and angering us to fight for health care issues as they specifically concern women. To do that means making connections among issues such as homophobia, racism, sexism, child care, and child rearing. AIDS magnifies the inequities of our social system. Fighting AIDS means increasing our own awareness of the connections between all social injustices. While we have to choose our battles based on localized or personalized considerations, it's important to keep thinking about all the complex connections that make up this struggle.

Activism and direct action take many forms. Writing a letter to the editor, leafletting at a shopping mall, setting up an information table outside a high school, coming out at work or to a family member are all forms of direct action that create change. Included here are various thoughts on our activism showing some of the personal developments of our politics; exploring issues around women, including lesbians, as AIDS activists; and touching on some of the barriers and inroads to our work. We also include an abridged outline of logistical and political considerations for creating actions and thoughts on evaluating our activism.

Considerations for Actions

Political Considerations

Target: Have a goal and determine strategy. Is it short or long term? Begin coalition building with another group or community to raise the public's awareness about, for example, getting a drug approved, more beds in a hospital, or nationalized health care. Some goals are more immediate than others. A short-term victory gives a lot of momentum for longer-term goals.

Also consider what makes an action successful. Putting up posters in a new neighborhood, handing out condoms outside a high school, guerrilla theater, publishing a letter to the editor, or having representatives on the radio or TV are all forms of direct action. Effectiveness is not limited to demonstrations and civil disobedience.

Each group must consider what it hopes to accomplish at that time and place. What risks (arrests, image, job loss, etc.) are there for members of the group? How do you create a balance so people feel safe as well as effective? How and when do you decide to "up the ante" by risking new things? What might the greater risks accomplish?

Coalitions/Working with Other Groups: Alliances and distance have their place. For instance, Gay Men's Health Crisis (GMHC) has gotten "respectability" out of the more "militant" image of ACT UP. The Association for Drug Abuse Prevention and Treatment (ADAPT) has also said that ACT UP "makes us look conservative." But also, there is great strength in working together on common goals, such as reproductive rights, prostitutes' rights, or advocacy for the homeless. In working in a coalition, or trying to develop one, it's important to learn to listen, share control, and accept as well as provide leadership. The type of action or scope of campaign might determine the balance of power between groups.

Racism/Classism in Activism: When considering risks (e.g., arrest situations), recognize that people have different relationships to the police based on experience, race, and class. For example, a white sex worker or a Black activist might choose not to participate in an action that could lead to arrest. Each community has diverse needs that require diverse responses. Do not make assumptions about risks or needs; rather, ask and listen, then build strategies that respect these differences.

Logistical Concerns/Doing a Demonstration

Concepts:

- Goal—what you want from the target.
- Target—whom/what action is for/against.
- Audience—whom are you trying to reach? For example, passersby, coworkers, media, politicians, community.
- Message—what do you want to say?
- Tactic—how will you achieve goal? Hit target? Reach audience? Get message across?

Logistics:

- When—time and date, including length of action. Consider "optimum people time" (when folks can be there) versus "optimum media time" (when the media can be there, e.g., live at 6 p.m.) versus "appropriate time" (opening bell on the stock exchange, when school lets out, changing of shifts at hospital, etc.).
- Where—location must be scouted beforehand. Outside: physical layout, space for picket, entrance/exits, photo opportunities, visibility to pedestrians, traffic, nearness to "target," security (yours and theirs). Inside: open to public? Layout, private versus public property.
- Publicity—getting people, as well as getting the word out. Organizing and mobilizing, as well as media work, press releases, phone calls, and so on.

Visuals/Themes:

- Communicating the message "Why we're here." Chants, puppets, posters, fact sheets, briefing people so anyone can be a spokesperson.

Tactics:

- Type of action—symbolic protest, disruption/interference, education/outreach, civil disobedience. (Remember arrests can be planned—that is, you plan on getting arrested—or unplanned— that is, the police arrest you because they feel like it. Know that this is not always something you can control.)

- Contingencies—"What if"...you can't get preferred spot? group is much larger or smaller than planned? weather is terrible? police presence not what you expected? initial demands met prior to the demonstration?
- Ending demonstration—deciding when to leave (fatigue, police harassment, goal achieved, point of diminished returns). Closing statement or gesture.

Follow-up and evaluation:

- *Any* change can make a demonstration a success. It might be in the form of a higher commitment in the group; renewed or increased enthusiasm; publicity for the issues; or a policy change, public apology, or change in position. Demonstrations and direct action are *tactics*—if you disrupt an office in an attempt to get a meeting with officials, you might want to use different tactics once you get the meeting. Also, discuss how you will follow up on demands. If your goal was to get a clinic to provide all clients with information on drug trials and how to get into them, how will you check to see that they are doing it? Ask to see the information they are giving to clients, or make helping to write the information part of your demand. Also, if the target agrees to your demand, let them know they did the right thing.
- Finally, what was the effect of the action on your group? How were people feeling about it at different points during the event? When offering or taking criticism, keep in mind that you and your coactivists are *on the same side*. Make it safe to criticize as well as praise each other and watch out for any "divide and conquer" possibilities.

Acknowledgments

The "Logistical Concerns/Doing a Demonstration" section is excerpted from a "Zap Outline" put together by Amy Bauer.

Focusing on Women: Video as Activism

JEAN CARLOMUSTO

When I first started working for Gay Men's Health Crisis (GMHC) in late 1986, the impact of AIDS on women was just beginning to be acknowledged. Although women had been dying of AIDS since at least 1981, this was denied by the press, media, and government until 1986. Following this blackout of information there was a media blitz of misinformation. The best way to tackle this situation was to get involved with a group actively doing work around women's issues. Through working with the Women's Caucus of ACT UP, I began to learn about direct action. This knowledge presented an urgent challenge to me as a videomaker to create direct action videotapes that focused on women's issues.

This experience continues to be valuable for me at GMHC and in other video AIDS activist groups in which I participate, such as Testing the Limits Collective and DIVA TV (Damned Interfering Video Activists). In contrast to network television, AIDS activist television explores the possibility of production within the context of an AIDS activist movement. Our videotapes are an effective way to share knowledge and strategies. Some of the formats we use in video production are direct action, grassroots educational, and militant eroticism video. As video activists our tapes are sometimes considered "raw." We make videos on extremely low budgets and get them out quickly. They are videotapes made in crisis mode.

Representing the political activity around the AIDS crisis entails taking on the politics of mainstream media. An example of the type of dangerous misinformation aimed at women in the mainstream media was an article in the January 1988 issue of *Cosmopolitan* magazine. This article, "Reassuring News about AIDS: A Doctor Tells Why You May Not Be At Risk" by Robert Gould, informed *Cosmo* readers that heterosexual women were not at risk for AIDS through "normal" heterosexual intercourse. A group of lesbians who had begun meeting socially within ACT UP read this article and decided to take direct action. Maria Maggenti and I collaborated on a tape about this action called *Doctors, Liars and Women: AIDS Activists Say No to Cosmo.*

Doctors, Liars and Women gives a genesis of the making of a demonstration. The process of making the videotape is discussed throughout the tape. We show a group of women from ACT UP's Women's Caucus confronting Dr. Gould with the information that the "evidence" in his article was not only out of date, but also incorrect. By challenging his authority with our knowledge, we make it clear that we are the experts. We also show how the demonstration at *Cosmopolitan's* office was organized and how the subsequent media coverage was dealt with. The goal of *Doctors, Liars and Women* is to inspire and demystify the process of doing direct action.

Women and AIDS is an example of educational grassroots video activism, for and about women. Alexandra Juhasz and I produced this tape for GMHC's "Living With AIDS" show on cable. *Women and AIDS* was made to educate women at risk, those working with women, and those concerned with women's issues. As in *Doctors, Liars and Women,* women are the only experts in this tape. The entire tape consists of interviews with them. These interviews range from interviews with workers at community-based organizations to candid "on the street" interviews. The goal of *Women and AIDS* is to give an overview of the issues that women face in the AIDS crisis.

Gregg Bordowitz and I began working on a series of safer-sex videos for GMHC in 1989. The purpose of the *Safer Sex Shorts* was to get the message out that safer sex can be hot. The format of these tapes blended advertisement, music video, and pornography into short pieces under five minutes in length. Task groups chose the situations and acts that were to be performed. Denise Ribble (a lesbian health educator and nurse who worked with PWAs at the Community Health Project in New York City) and I designed one for women who have sex with women. The recognition of lesbian sexuality, as well as the Centers for Disease Control's persistent refusal to include data on woman-to-woman transmission, were the primary motivations in creating the lesbian safer-sex video *Current Flow.*

Lesbian-identified sex-positive imagery is scarce. This is both oppressive and dangerous, because in order to educate lesbians about safer sex we have to establish what safer sex for lesbians is. Saying "use a dental dam" is not the same as saying "use a condom" since many women don't even know what a dental dam is. So, we

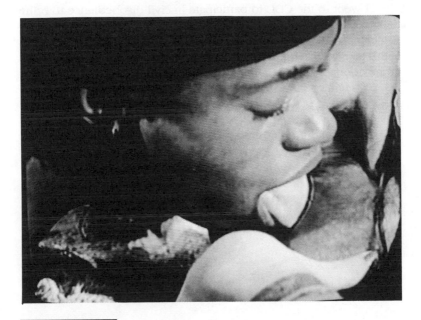

Shara and Annie demonstrate their dexterity with a dental dam in "Current Flow," a lesbian safe-sex video from Gay Men's Health Crisis Safer Sex Shorts Series.

Video still by Jean Carlomusto.

showed how to use a dental dam and latex gloves by having two women graphically demonstrate on my couch. That's what direct action video is about.

As I write this piece, I have just returned from the Centers for Disease Control (CDC) in Atlanta. ACT UP organized a protest and civil disobedience to abolish the outmoded and unscientific definitions of AIDS and to revise the epidemiological methods of the CDC. I was part of an affinity group called the "Condams" (a better way of saying dental dam). Our specific focus was how the CDC's definitions of AIDS exclude the kind of opportunistic infections that affect women. Conditions such as chlamydia, pelvic inflammatory disease, and papilloma virus become life threatening when combined with HIV. These conditions aren't classified as AIDS by the CDC.

The Condams wore T-shirts that had vaginas and uteruses on them with logos saying "Unknown Zone," "Sexism = Death," and "The CDC Ignores Women." We staged a "die-in" in front of the door of the CDC.

I went to the CDC to participate in civil disobedience to bring to light that after nine years of the AIDS crisis, women are still being neglected and ignored by the health care and social services systems in this country. Up until the moment I lay down on the ground in front of the doors of the CDC, I had a video camera in my hands.

We will continue to fight until the AIDS crisis is over.

To get any of the tapes described here, contact: GMHC Videotapes/Publications Distribution, 129 W. 20th St., New York, NY 10011. See also "AIDS Videos By, For, and About Women" on page 281 of this book.

Talking that Talk

DIANA DIANA

*A vibrant grassroots program, the South Carolina AIDS Educa-
tion Network (SCAEN) operates primarily out of DiAna's Hair Ego, the
director's hair salon. Here, condoms are piled next to curlers, and
clients view AIDS videos while getting their hair done. In a state with
some of the most restrictive and punitive HIV laws and a reactionary
political climate, people are hungry for information that respects their
lives. This program operates on the commitment of its activist volunteers, without state support, and offers critical peer education to the
Black community. Outreach has spilled out of the salon into
churches, schools, and other community forums. SCAEN's strategy is
to confront AIDS and sex in realistic ways, whether it's through
conducting safe-sex "Tupperware" parties for adults, or having kids
produce a coloring book for other kids on the fears and facts of AIDS.*

My name is DiAna DiAna. I am President and Executive Director
of the South Carolina AIDS Education Network, Inc. (SCAEN). We
incorporated in November 1987. My partner, Dr. Bambi Sumpter, has
a doctorate in public health from the University of South Carolina in
the area of human sexuality and family life education. She is SCAEN's
Director of Youth Services. We have worked together for the past few
years and have trained nearly 10,000 people in South Carolina. We do
that in many different ways—doing AIDS presentations in schools,
churches, civic groups, and women's groups. We also do education
of children; we even get to do them outside (we really do *grass* roots,
you know, get barefoot, and get down on the grass with the children
and talk that talk!). Bambi and I have developed our own educational
materials; we have coloring books for the kids, and a low-reading
reader for the people who can't read well—that is a big problem here
in South Carolina.

We once did an NAACP group outside in the park and we had about 73 people, about 20 of them kids ten years and under. Bambi talked to the kids and we gave out all the flyers for the teens, and all the coloring books, and then I gave out the low-reading books. A Black woman came up to me and asked for one of the flyers; I offered her some of the adult material I had and she said "no," she said that she wanted the "other kind of book." She pointed to the "low reader" that one of the passing kids had, and I told her that we didn't have any left. She just looked out at the sky and started to bite her lip, and she got tears in her eyes. I offered to mail her some but she said "no." I realized that she could not read and probably didn't want anyone to know. The few flyers we had were copies that some of my beauty shop clients had made for me in their offices. We operate from clients' funds, donations, and "a little help from my friends." That day was the first time that I felt how strong the need was for us to try to do more and to do better.

It was my clients who first brought to my attention that people had already been quarantined in a nearby community. I tried to tell as many people about it as I could, but that was still not enough. I started to circulate petitions to request ACT UP to come to South Carolina to help expose the problem. In April 1989 that wish came true. Although ACT UP didn't have much visual support…reason being that the demonstration was played down by the media, and people who worked for some of the state agencies were told that if they came out to show support their job might be in danger. But anyway, after ACT UP left, everyone knew about the quarantine and everyone had become more aware of the AIDS problem here. I personally would like to thank them for helping us.

I have written four plays. The one called "Dad Remember When…" is about prom night and what the kids do to get ready; then they get a hotel room and go from there. The play is currently being performed by the students at Allen University. I am very proud of all the students. They come to rehearsal faithfully twice a week from 8:45 'til 10:30. They do not get paid, and they have performed the play seven times to large audiences. Allen University has given us the full use of their theater and we invite other students to come in and watch the play. The first scene the teacher does is "AIDS 101" and the audience loves it. We have as many onlookers as we do performers. The kids have asked me when do we start the other AIDS play so they can try out for parts. The kids take what they have learned and tell their friends. They talk to their friends in their own language so that they understand each other. I hope someone recognizes all the talent

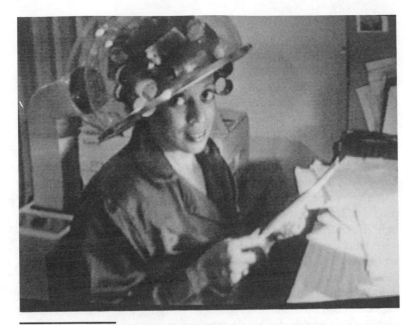

DiAna DiAna, catching up on SCAEN's correspondence. Still from "DiAna's Hair Ego: AIDS Info Up Front."
Videotape by Ellen Spiro.

we have in our youths and makes good use of it. It works!!

People keep saying why don't we get funded. Well, one reason is I work a full-time job and so does my partner. The other part is I have been told that I have "questionable" credentials. I admit I don't have a Ph.D. I only have an associate's degree in child care, and I am just a cosmetologist, but Bambi and I were both trained under DHEC (the Department of Health and Environmental Control). We filed reports that gave DHEC their needed statistics for training minorities, but they never agreed to support us in turn. When we stopped giving them reports, we became "questionable."

For the past three years I have financed SCAEN through my Mastercharge and through my clients' tips from the beauty shop, and through donations that Bambi and I have received for doing presentations on AIDS. SCAEN is solely financed "by the people," because we are for the people. The very fact that we have been able to survive this long on "nothing" means that we are worth "something." Bambi and I are the only two staff people in the program. We own it, and operate it, and design all the programs, and codirect the plays, and write the literature. We do have more volunteers than you can imagine. Most of the volunteers are women that come from the beauty salon and see the materials that I have displayed in the shop and they ask us to come out into the community to do the presentations. They bring their children into the shop to watch the AIDS videos that I show during the day, and I welcome them to ask any questions that they might have. The kids feel comfortable talking to me and so do their parents.

The statistics here in South Carolina keep going up higher and higher and it seems no end is in sight. People must understand that when you can't talk about sex and you can't use the "condom word" on TV, it is really difficult to educate people. The "powers that be" here in South Carolina must recognize that there are a lot of people here who cannot read, so putting up another poster isn't going to work. You have to get out and talk with people. You must answer all their questions, and take the time to make sure that they understand you. You cannot place "your old tired morals" on today's youths and expect to communicate. Everything is changing, and you must change with it if you expect the next generation to survive. Bambi and I have decided that we will keep on working as long as we are wanted...besides, money isn't everything, money isn't everything. Money isn't everything...if I keep saying it I might even believe it.

The South Carolina AIDS Education Network can be contacted at Suite 98, 2768 Decker Blvd., Columbia, SC 29206 (803) 736-1171. Their Safer-Sex Kit ($35) contains a Safer-Sex User Guide, condoms, spermicide, dental dams, finger cots, a vibrator, and other items.

We Have a Job to Do

BAMBI SUMPTER

Sometimes finding the right path in the midst of a storm can turn out to be a frustrating, yet spiritual experience. As you stumble amidst turbulent winds and rain, flying objects, and a general atmosphere of uncertainty, you wonder about the probability that you will survive. Yet, somehow you know that you are a survivor. That you are capable of creating a solution to your dilemma. You begin to persevere, to demonstrate your tenacity…out of a basic need to survive, you muster up all that your spirit can…you have transcended!

The South Carolina AIDS Education Network, Inc. (SCAEN) is only another grassroots organization that is attempting to fight the AIDS epidemic amidst turbulent winds and many periods of uncertainty. We are not special, for we know of many organizations which continue to survive the bureaucratic rhetoric, personal vendettas, and the egos of those who hold purse strings, intimidated by the ingenuity of people who lack a plethora of bachelor, masters, and doctoral degrees. Let us say there is "grave" concern over the "credentials" of those who are delivering the AIDS message.

I was privileged to meet DiAna DiAna during an AIDS "Train the Trainer" workshop. At that time it was our false assumption that the purpose of such training was to create a mechanism to reach out to the community and educate them about this devastating disease. As the years passed since that training, we have come to the realization that the AIDS epidemic is the most political and economic issue of our time.

We have realized that, be it conscious or unconscious, the "overseers" attempt to dictate who will deliver the message and, of course, it will be by their rules and direction. Ignorance to cultural differences abounds. We have come to understand that although the "powers that be" understand the devastation that awaits our generation, politically they are unprepared for and/or unwilling to do what is necessary.

In the past two years, there has been a 40 percent increase in HIV/AIDS infection among adolescents. Despite this figure, political factions continue to deny the existence of thousands of sexually active teens, runaways, and throwaways, at risk for HIV infection. They refuse to acknowledge the danger in not providing behavior-specific education to a population of young people who are constantly bombarded with messages promoting sexual activity without protection.

Our organization has provided a variety of services to the community. From January 1987 until the present we have provided one-to-one AIDS information to over 9,000 individuals in South Carolina. SCAEN updates information as it becomes available. Information is requested from organizations throughout the nation and world. This information is utilized to enhance the effectiveness of public AIDS workshops, as well as teacher training.

Delivery of services takes from one hour to several days, depending on need. Follow-up services are part of the educational groups. AIDS education videos are shown daily at DiAna's Hair Ego Salon in Columbia, South Carolina. AIDS pamphlets and materials are given to customers, and mini-seminars are held in the shop during the day. The development of special AIDS education materials that are specifically geared for youth, from kindergarten children to older adolescents, is a major priority. Materials are also geared to consider the poor or nonreader.

The major focus of SCAEN activities is to create opportunities in which members of the community can actively participate in educating themselves about AIDS. A $50 poster contest for young people served as the mechanism to develop one of SCAEN's more popular brochures, as well as a coloring book for kids and a booklet for nonreaders.

DiAna created MAA, which stands for Mothers Against AIDS. MAA is a support group for mothers and fathers who need to know what is really happening with their children, and what they are doing. The formation of this group provides an opportunity for parents to exchange stories, learn to help each other cope with the challenges of parenting, as well as learn about the disease. Apathy and fear have strongly affected the success of this group, but efforts will continue to raise the consciousness of parents. SCAEN presently has a weekly column in a local community newspaper, *The Carolina Panorama*. The column seeks to address issues related to AIDS and how the individual reader can apply the information in their life.

SCAEN provides a service for adults 18 years of age and older called "AIDS 102: Saving Lives Through Prevention—Safe-Sex Program." The primary goal of AIDS 102 is to engage the participants in noncontact activities, desensitize them in order to create a learning environment, promote the ideals of abstinence and sexual responsibility as options, and guide the participants in the creation of their very own specific *safe-sex* behaviors or alternatives to reduce the likelihood of infection. We now have the "Safer-Sex Kit" on the mail-order market. This behavior-change kit will provide AIDS educators with a tool to teach safer sexual practices which reduce the likelihood of HIV/AIDS infection, as well as provide protection for any sexually active person who cares about their life and the lives of their partners.

To date, our funding has come from the salon's client tips and the donations of community people who understand our cause. Despite all of our attempts, programs, and successes, it has been decided by the "powers" that SCAEN is unworthy of funding. We "lack grant-writing expertise." "We cannot fund everyone who asks for funds" is one favorite and famous phrase. Finally, "your management procedures leave much to be desired." Given that SCAEN has gone through the scrutiny necessary to become a nonprofit, tax-exempt organization, it seems funny that the Department of Health would see a problem with our management style. I wonder how many lives have become affected by HIV while they ponder and wallow in the aforementioned concerns? We are willing to work along with the "powers," but they too must be prepared to respect us for our expertise and knowledge of strategies to promote behavior change, especially in the minority community.

SCAEN, Inc., is grateful for the opportunity to express our concerns. We are deeply grateful to ACT UP for their emotional support while we try to save lives. We appreciate the support of the National AIDS Network in sponsoring us to attend their Skills Building Workshops. Without their help we would have difficulty networking and staying in contact with our allies. We appreciate the support of those churches that understand that God intends for us to reach out to all of our brothers and sisters, regardless of age, color, culture, sexual identity, or socioeconomic status. Without a doubt, SCAEN, Inc. has transcended! We will not turn around…we have a job to do…and no one can prevent us from saving lives! We have and will continue to weather the storm…with or without the financial backing of the bureaucracy…Thanks Be To God!

Facing Reality:
AIDS Education and Women of Color

DAZON DIXON

I knew when I chose to work on women's health from the AIDS perspective that I was facing a real challenge. But I never expected anything as difficult as the reality of what conquering this epidemic (without a cure) is truly going to take.

I entered the field of AIDS education very deliberately and with much forethought. As an African-American feminist educator on women's health issues, it was pressing and vital that I participate in AIDS in this way. Health care and social service agencies were finally beginning to recognize and count positive-diagnosed women as persons living with AIDS, and the numbers were beginning to rise. Direct outreach to women was not yet commonplace. Our safer-sex workshops and "Do It Safe" parties were innovative, fresh, and effective. At the time, I thought that we were on the true cutting edge, that we were making time to prevent AIDS from spreading too far into any population of women.

Was I ever wrong! The edge keeps slipping farther away, and the numbers of women who are becoming infected and sick and dying are continuing to rise. To exacerbate the problem for me, African-American women stand to suffer tremendously from the AIDS epidemic. It is not enough to know that women of color are at greatest risk of becoming affected by AIDS. We all need to constantly know that African-American women are still at the bottom of the economic ladder in the United States. Black women endure more violence within our communities and relationships, are subject to more crimes, are more vulnerable to the drug epidemic, have poorer health care, survive more rape and incest experiences, have fewer sexual and reproductive health choices, and die faster of most terminal diseases. Our lifestyles, particularly our relationships with men and drugs, are killing us. For many of us, living with or without AIDS, this is reality.

As an educator and an activist on women's health and AIDS issues, this is what I must face—for myself and for those with whom I share my service.

There are some definite points of reality to the effect of AIDS. We know that over half the cases in women are in Black women. And that 80 percent of the cases in children are in babies born to women of color. We should know that AIDS is the fastest growing killer among women of childbearing age, particularly young women of color—ahead of diabetes, influenza, and pneumonia. AIDS is the fifth leading cause of death among Black women.

These, however, are just *some* of the facts that can be described with numbers. These women are the ones they counted. What about the other truths (the less visible to the "average" eye) that some would rather leave unaddressed? For example, Black women die faster after AIDS diagnosis than anyone else; more women are dying never having had an AIDS diagnosis; health care is so atrocious (particularly for indigent patients) that many of us are dying without any care. Women are dying in places where they have no name and no voice. Their families, if present, are stigmatized and ostracized, left to deal with the disease even after it has destroyed the family's primary caregiver.

Knowing all these truths, how impactful can I be on a group of women who are more into survival than living? Seeing the universal effects of racism, sexism, classism, ableism, ageism, and homophobia directly and indirectly killing people, am I to go on giving out condoms and safety squares (dental dams) and ideas on erotic safe sex as the solution? Is it really feasible for me to discuss sexual behavior change when people are not even in touch with their sexual behavior? Having a firm grasp on what the real challenge of preventing the spread of AIDS is about, do I have the courage, the strength, and ability to take it all on?

I know that I do not have all the answers to my questions. I do know that I am committed to working toward eradicating the scourge of AIDS in our communities. Since I began my work in AIDS, I have revisited many times the dream of beating the spread of this disease with brainpower, self-empowerment, and spiritual clarity. We should be able to out-think a virus and prevent it from destroying lives.

AIDS is forcing us all to reexamine our sexual and general health priorities. It has opened a gigantic Pandora's box of the social ills and oppression that women of color are surviving. Now we are seeing the Western-white-male-dominated culture behave in its true form. In the name of investment and profit, poor health care planning, and lack of interest in the affected lives, they are watching people die.

As AIDS continues its journey through vulnerable lives, we all will find challenges to change our attitudes. For women of color, however, particularly African-American women, it is much more than an attitude. We need to evaluate our lifestyle choices and choose those activities and relationships that make sense for our health, for our families, and most importantly, for ourselves. We need to be clear that no situation or condition is isolated from others. If we are victims of poverty, violence, drug infiltration, hate, neglect, disrespect, ignorance, and an overwhelming lack of support, then we are the most vulnerable people to AIDS. We must recognize how our choices help us participate in taking unnecessary risks. We must face our realities and keep them in the perspective of our life situations. We must work to change—to stop surviving and start living. I am convinced that is the best method of prevention.

About the Author

Dázon Dixon coordinates Sisterlove Women's AIDS Project in Atlanta, Georgia.

Changing the Whole Approach

GAIL HARRIS

Women are at risk for HIV and AIDS because they don't recognize themselves in standard prevention and education campaigns. A major obstacle to education is sexism—dealing with women as a preconceived group—with no attempt to focus on women as individuals, without understanding how women live. Another major obstacle is racism, which manifests itself in policies directed towards a particular subgroup within the HIV community, as with intravenous drug users (IVDUs) in New York and Miami. These data are used to portray all women with AIDS as women of color and IVDUs.

If you hear me being a skeptic—I am that. I'm tired of the posturing; if this is a crisis of the proportions spoken of by the World Health Organization and the Centers for Disease Control, why is the response so poor? Let educational intervention get as explicit as necessary. There's so much being spent having people sit in rooms regurgitating facts to make them "palatable." And then I get calls from women who are HIV positive living in the boonies, "Please send me everything you have on AIDS." What do we have that's helpful, explicit, and understandable to send?

To change this situation, women must first be recognized as valuable human beings, not as vectors of infection. Then we need to have the resources, the professional facilities, and the technical and financial organization that men have. Women need the same level of support that men get: corporate concern that is woman centered.

What I'm talking about is no less than a whole revolution in our way of seeing this crisis and in the way women are perceived. It's difficult to maintain an identity in this crisis. Women are viewed in their roles as "partners of..." or viewed as bearers of children. I know who I am, yet there's a point at which I still don't see any identifiable resources to plug into. This makes for insanity. I'm disappointed that the reproductive rights movement didn't see a need to broaden itself to look at women's health as a whole.

Organizing something like a women's health institute could mean creating for many women the only time and place they get some level of consideration. Why not broaden it and make it more specific at the same time: adolescent health emphasized as *female* adolescent health. The only adolescents I know who are getting pregnant are female. Education must become supportive, must provide an environment where people can admit their ignorances, learn, and move on. We need early intervention, including behavioral strategies, to challenge women's health risks in the areas of sexual health and AIDS.

About the Author

Gail Harris now works with the Center for Women's Policy Studies (CWPS) in Washington, D.C. As a member of the Brooklyn AIDS Task Force she became involved in video production, seeing the connections between the visual arts as education and the specific needs of AIDS education. She has been an artist-in-residence at Downtown Community Television in New York, and has organized screenings of AIDS and safer-sex tapes. In 1988 the CWPS established the National Resource Center on Women and AIDS as a central clearinghouse for both policymakers and activists engaged in prevention education and policy development around AIDS.

AIDS and Politics: Transformation of Our Movement

MAXINE WOLFE

Over most of the 30 years of my political activism, I was somehow always on the "periphery of the periphery." The question, then, is: "How could a nice Jewish girl from Brooklyn, who once described herself as a bisexual, Trotskyist, anarchist, Reichian, lesbian-feminist, end up in an organization people continually describe as white, male, bourgeois (worse yet, upper middle class), single issue, not gay identified, arrogant, resource rich, and every other thing that people who describe themselves as 'progressive' don't like?" The second question is: "Why have I stayed in it?"

I came to AIDS activism and to New York ACT UP out of a queer consciousness, a consciousness forced on me by the sexism and homophobia of the male-identified left in this country and by the homophobia of the women's movement. I came to ACT UP because of the inability of lesbians to organize around or even figure out what their issues were and because of the dead end of the "identity" politics of the early 1980s.

I had joined the reproductive rights movement in 1978 to organize against the elimination of Medicaid funding for abortion, after I had left the Trotskyist group—whose periphery I had been on for several years. They disparagingly called the reproductive rights group which I joined "feminist," but I said I would rather argue for my Marxist politics in a feminist group than for my feminist politics in a Marxist group. Five years later, in 1984, I decided I'd rather do neither. And by that time I had decided I didn't want to be in a lesbian-feminist group, and I didn't want to be in a lesbian and gay left group. What had happened?

Some of the things these groups had in common were an outdated concept of organizing, an unwillingness to reach outside their known constituencies, and a rigid set of politics around which

AIDS and Politics 233

everyone had to agree. Then you couldn't question anything or you were suspect.

Identity politics had gotten to the point where, apparently, the only person I was supposed to feel comfortable talking to was another working-class, Jewish, lesbian mother of two children from the left who was neither vanilla nor chocolate. Everybody was in their own separate box and I didn't have a box to fit into.

By 1984, I was severely depressed. All of the groups I had worked with since 1979 no longer existed. I was forced to reevaluate every political perspective and value I ever had. I started going to every meeting I could find, including lesbian and gay Democrats. I decided I had to clear out my head of previous indoctrination, really listen to what people said, and really look at what they were doing.

I did a range of different things between 1984 and 1987, but three stand out. First, I began my still-weekly treks as a volunteer to the Lesbian Herstory Archives, the only remaining woman-only space in New York, where a truly diverse group of women work together, committed to preserving the full range of lesbian experience. But it was not enough for my activist bones. Second, I went to the first public meeting of the Gay and Lesbian Alliance Against Defamation and saw that at least 400 gay men and a few lesbians wanted to do activist work around homophobia and AIDS. I didn't join, however, because their operating style was the familiar "progressive" model. In addition, in response to my questions, one of their answers was that they were neither for nor against the closing of the bathhouses. That turned me off. I was against the closing of the bathhouses. The third significant event (or rather, events) were the Hardwick demonstrations after the Supreme Court upheld Georgia's antigay sodomy law—both the spontaneous sit-in of hundreds one night in Sheridan Square and the several thousand who, four days later on July 4th, marched into the throngs of tourists at the Statue of Liberty Centennial against the desires of the self-appointed "gay leadership." I realized that the community was ahead of its so-called "leadership" and willing to put their bodies on the line at the right moment. This gave me hope.

Almost one year later, a week before the Lesbian and Gay Pride March in 1987, a friend of mine told me about an AIDS activist group. As if by fate, at the march I saw this guy selling "Silence = Death" T-shirts. I went over to him and asked, "Are there women in your group?" "Sure," he said. So the next evening I found myself at the Lesbian and Gay Community Center in a group of a couple of hundred men I didn't know and about four women.

Why did I stay when, in terms of political perspective, many things about this group should have told me to leave? For example, I had assumed it was a lesbian- and gay-identified group, but people didn't want to be called lesbian and gay activists; they wanted to be called "AIDS activists." And they seemed to believe in the health care system, even if it had gone awry. They even respected doctors!

But everything was run democratically, and people got up and said what they thought. I could get up and say what I thought. They wanted to end the AIDS crisis, period, and if you had a good idea they would listen. No one spouted rhetoric; there was no party line. They had great ideas for actions without any pre-set idea of the right way to do things. They thought tabling was a new idea. They had a great sense of the visual and they used the media, but they didn't cater to it. No one quibbled over words on a flyer. If you wanted to do an action, you proposed it. Most likely people would do it. In fact, they did more actions in a week than I'd ever thought possible. And they have made more of an impact, both conceptually and in terms of saving people's lives, than any group I've ever been part of. These were people organizing not from some abstract concept but to save their lives and the lives of people they cared about. And, they were pro-sex at a time when sex was being connected to death.

But I am a realist and not a romantic. I don't think ACT UP is the be-all and end-all. There have been problems. I stayed in ACT UP because it is a place where I can be a lesbian, a woman, and an activist. I stayed in ACT UP because I have seen people *develop* a political perspective, including myself. I have changed and learned or I wouldn't still be there. It is also the first real organizing I feel I've ever done. I have seen men who wanted to hide being gay behind their AIDS activism do a teach-in on lesbian and gay history, become more and more openly gay, and develop a gay liberation, and not a gay rights, perspective. I have seen the issues expand—a year ago no one talked about nationalized health care; now we have a national health care committee and are talking to unions about doing an action together. ACT UP is a true coalition. Everyone puts up with what my mother would call everyone else's *mischigas*—craziness. I have come to appreciate what each person can and will contribute because they share a commitment to the saving of lives.

I no longer feel like I'm on the periphery of the periphery. For the first time, I feel I am acting from my center but not from the mainstream. I feel I'm helping to build a movement that is mine rather than trying to fit into someone else's.

I don't know where ACT UP will go. Your guess is as good as mine. As for our movement, the lesbian and gay and AIDS movement,

I believe that in order to take advantage of the momentum for the future, we need to seriously check out our own homophobia and our rigid rules for evaluating political movements. This is especially true for older lesbians and for lesbians and gay men who identify with progressive movements. For example, there are two questions I am always asked by lesbians who look down on AIDS work, and by lesbians and gay men working in other progressive movements. One is: "Would gay men have done the same thing for lesbians if the situation had been reversed?" The first thing I say is, "I am not in this movement for gay men; I am in this movement for myself." And then I ask them: "What have straight women and straight men done for us? What have the antinuclear and anti-intervention movements done for us?" I'm not saying that people shouldn't work in these movements. I am saying, "Check out the homophobia in your question." The second question I am asked is: "If a cure for AIDS happened tomorrow, wouldn't all those gay men go home and not care about access issues?" "Probably a lot would," I answer, "just like all the women who went home after *Roe v. Wade* and only came out again when *Roe* was threatened." The fact is that poor women—and because of institutional racism in this country, Black and Latin women are disproportionately among the poor—and young women and rural women have not had access to abortion for many, many years. Where were these women in 1977 when the Hyde Amendment, cutting off federal Medicaid funding for abortion, was passed? Gay men, as a group, are no better and no worse than anyone else. We have to get past this mentality.

In that respect, one of the most important roles that ACT UP plays is that it is a place where many younger gay men and lesbians have come to understand that what we want is the right to exist—not the right to privacy; the right to a life, not to a lifestyle; and a life that is as important as anyone else's, but not any more important than anyone else's. This understanding has formed the basis for work outside of the lesbian and gay community, with other communities affected by the AIDS crisis, and it is why ACT UP has been managing to do some of that work.

Many younger lesbians in ACT UP see themselves as "queer," and both their political and social life is tied to that of gay men. While I have made good gay male and lesbian friends in ACT UP, many of whom will remain my friends for a long time, ACT UP does not satisfy my social needs. But I am not into coupledom or monogamy in my political life any more than in my social life. ACT UP is my political home for now. And, I can honestly say that while in 1979 there were only a handful of gay men in New York I could work with politically, after ACT UP, there will be more. That's not bad.

This is an edited version of a speech presented at the National Gay and Lesbian Task Force Town Meeting, October 6, 1989, in Washington, D.C.

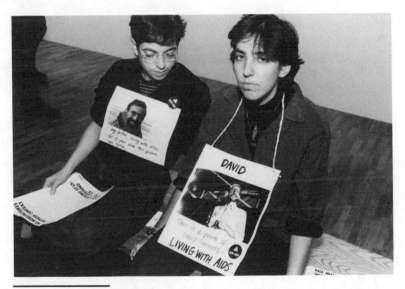

Activists at the opening of "Nicholas Nixon: Pictures of People" at the Museum of Modern Art in New York in September, 1988, protesting morbid photographs and calling for less objectifying, more empowering images of PWAs.

Photo by T. L. Litt

The Denver Principles

The Denver Principles[1] were drawn up at the second AIDS Forum, held in Denver in 1983, where the National Association of People with AIDS was formed. This "manifesto of self-empowerment" [2] served to let it be known that PWAs were taking control of their lives and of how they would be treated by the medical establishment and by the public. They would not accept the label of victims and the passivity that implies. While a milestone document, this does not address many of the specific needs and demands of women PWAs. We look forward to a similar manifesto that will. —The Book Group

We condemn attempts to label us as "victims," which implies defeat, and we are only occasionally "patients," which implies passivity, helplessness, and dependence upon the care of others. We are "people with AIDS."

We recommend that health care professionals

1. Who are gay, come out, especially to their patients who have AIDS.

2. Always clearly identify and discuss the theory they favor as to the cause of AIDS, since this bias affects the treatment and advice they give.

3. Get in touch with their feelings (fears, anxieties, hopes, etc.) about AIDS, and not simply deal with AIDS intellectually.

4. Take a thorough personal inventory and identify and examine their own agendas around AIDS.

5. Treat people with AIDS as whole people and address psychosocial issues as well as biophysical ones.

6. Address the question of sexuality in people with AIDS specifically, sensitively, and with information about gay male sexuality in general and the sexuality of people with AIDS in particular.

We recommend that all people

1. Support us in our struggle against those who would fire us from our jobs, evict us from our homes, refuse to touch us, separate us from our loved ones, our community, or our peers, since there is no evidence that AIDS can be spread by casual social contact.

2. Do not scapegoat people with AIDS, blame us for the epidemic, or generalize about our lifestyles.

We recommend that people with AIDS

1. Form caucuses to choose their own representatives, to deal with the media, to choose their own agenda, and to plan their own strategies.

2. Be involved at every level of AIDS decision making and specifically serve on the boards of directors of provider organizations.

3. Be included in all AIDS forums with equal credibility as other participants, to share their own experiences and knowledge.

4. Substitute low-risk sexual behaviors for those that could endanger themselves or their partners, and we feel that people with AIDS have an ethical responsibility to inform their potential sexual partners of their health status.

People with AIDS have the right

1. To as full and satisfying sexual and emotional lives as anyone else.

2. To quality medical treatment and quality social service provision, without discrimination in any form, including sexual orientation, gender, diagnosis, economic status, age, or race.

3. To full explanations of all medical procedures and risks, to choose or refuse their treatment modalities, to refuse to participate in research without jeopardizing their treatment, and to make informed decisions about their lives.

4. To privacy, to confidentiality of medical records, to human respect, and to choose who their significant others are.

5. To die and *live* in dignity.

Notes

1. The PWA Coalition *Newsline,* no. 1, June 1985.
2. Mike Navarre, "Fighting the Victim Label: PWA Coalition Portfolio," *AIDS: Cultural Analysis/Cultural Activism,* Douglas Crimp, ed. (Cambridge: MIT Press, 1988), pp. 144-145.

Conclusion

The AIDS crisis—and the recent threats to hard-won reproductive rights—have revived the forms of direct action used in the civil rights, feminist, and gay liberation movements as strategies for political change. But you don't have to shout at a government building and get arrested to be an activist. Activism on many issues can take many forms. Informally exchanging safer-sex information in a conversation with a friend, or pointing out the bigotry in a colleague's remarks, or questioning what you hear on the news from a government official, for example, are all forms of activism. All that is required is that you are angry about the lack of information or services in your community and are willing to put yourself on the line in some way to make it change. It's easy enough, with the first little bits of information about AIDS, for example, to recognize lies and to realize you have a lot more accurate information than a lot of the self-proclaimed and societally instituted experts and professionals. As activists in the feminist health care movement said and AIDS activists are now saying, "We are the experts."

This book, for example, emerged from a common base of feminism and a common commitment to ending the AIDS crisis. We knew there was too little known about women in the crisis, particularly from an activist perspective. Some of us were already experts on some topics (like health care or drug use or safe sex), but none of us knew the specific answers to questions that were taking shape in our minds. Why do women die six times faster than men do after receiving an AIDS diagnosis? Why are women dying of HIV-related illnesses without receiving an AIDS diagnosis that would qualify them for certain treatments and benefits? How does HIV present itself differently in women's bodies? How have racism, sexism, and heterosexism prevented people from receiving adequate prevention information or adequate treatment? Why, a decade into the epidemic, do we still not have adequate information and services? How can we challenge what we are being told by the "authorities" in the government and the medical profession? What research isn't being done? What questions aren't *they* asking—and why? Writing this book was not simply a way to express what we already knew, but a way to find out what we didn't know and why this information was not available.

Women, AIDS, and Activism brings together many of the issues around the AIDS crisis as they affect women—not only practical information about how to prevent HIV transmission; about the personal and legal ramifications of an HIV-antibody test; and about diagnosis, treatment, and other medical issues for women, but also a confrontation of the institutionalized racism, sexism, and heterosexism that prevent people from getting the information and services they need. In addressing all these issues, one of our foremost goals was to promote activism as a way of responding to these issues.

But activism isn't easy. It requires a willingness to confront not only the ideology and bureaucracy of the government, the medical establishment, corporations, and the mass media, but also our own conditioned attitudes. Sexism within an organization, for example, or racism that prevents an organization from working in coalition with other organizations with similar goals, may be issues that are painful and time consuming to address, but there is no way to get done what we have to get done without doing so. AIDS is not a single-issue crisis and it's not an issue that is only of concern to people with AIDS. It affects all of us and is informed by every type of oppression. There is no one oppression that needs to be combated in order to end the AIDS crisis.

Racism, heterosexism, and sexism, particularly, haunt every attempt to build even transitory coalitions. But coalition building is not about diversity for its own sake. Often it requires working with a lot of people you may not completely agree with politically. Having lots of different people in the same group or in a coalition may make the work harder—but it is necessary to achieve our long-term goals. Already the AIDS activist movement and the reproductive rights movement have begun to recognize common goals; AIDS activists and those advocating for IV drug users have begun to work together around issues such as needle exchange; and universal access to health care is appearing on the agendas of many movements, from AIDS activism to labor union organizing. Failure to build coalitions has always contributed to our respective marginalization and invisibility.

In the AIDS crisis, women are most of the time completely invisible, face severe and sometimes insurmountable obstacles to coming out with a positive HIV status, have almost no research done about them, have little money, are rarely provided with adequate care, and have to take care of the most people. In the face of such dark shadows of indifference, ignorance, and antagonism, activism may in fact be the only hopeful and viable response—the difference between whether or not our health care system collapses and the determining structure for our future standards of survival.

Glossary

BRIGITTE WEIL

Ableism: the discriminatory practice of beliefs that consider that differently abled bodies are inherently inferior to abled bodies.

ACTG (AIDS Clinical Trials Group): system of cooperative medical institutions conducting NIAID's clinical AIDS drug trials.

ACT UP (AIDS Coalition to Unleash Power): a diverse nonpartisan group united in anger and committed to direct action to end the AIDS crisis. A group of concerned individuals outraged by the government's mismanagement of the AIDS crisis united to form ACT UP in New York City in March 1987.

AIDS (acquired immunodeficiency syndrome): a viral syndrome that impairs the body's ability to fight disease. The suppression of the immune system leads to a weakening of the body's defenses against a variety of infections, viruses, and malignancies.

AmFAR (American Foundation for AIDS Research): a private nonprofit organization founded by Mathilde Krim to fund research. Its very existence reveals the scandalous inadequacy of the federal response to the AIDS crisis.

Anemia: a condition that decreases the ability of red blood cells to deliver oxygen to the body.

Anonymous testing: the only kind of testing that respects and protects the privacy of an individual. In the case of testing for the antibodies to HIV, your blood sample is identified only by a number and the testing institution has no record of your name.

Antibody: a blood cell that recognizes and targets a specific invading substance.

Antigen: a substance that stimulates production of antibodies.

Antiviral: a substance that stops or suppresses the activity of a virus.

Approval: refers to the only process for distribution of drugs in the United States, according to law and FDA regulations. It involves the following six steps: (1) Preclinical—laboratory and animal studies; (2) Company files investigational new drug (IND) with FDA; (3) Clinical Phase I—testing for safety; Phase II—testing effectiveness of the dose and for the condition prescribed; Phase III—extensive clinical trials; (4) Company files new drug application with FDA; (5) FDA review; (6) FDA approval.

ARC (AIDS-related complex): a loose categorization of AIDS-related symptoms that are linked to HIV infection but are not included in the specific case definition of AIDS by the CDC. The differentiation between people with ARC and people with AIDS is significant because many social services, as well as health care, are dependent on an official AIDS diagnosis, and are not otherwise available to people with ARC, even though they might show serious disabling symptoms. A term in disfavor among AIDS activists, as it is understood to impose distinctions artificially among people with HIV-related illness, excluding HIV-positive people from much needed benefits and services.

Asymptomatic: infection without symptoms. Although you might test positive for HIV, you might not necessarily show symptoms of HIV infection.

Candida: a yeast organism that normally lives in the intestines but can flourish in other parts of the body during immunosuppression. When candida affects the mouth, it is called thrush.

CDC (U.S. Centers for Disease Control): federal agency of the Public Health Service whose mandate is to track the incidence and trends of communicable diseases and also certain noninfectious diseases. Its responsibilities include disease surveillance, licensing of clinical laboratories, conducting research, and training epidemiologists and health workers. For the latest CDC figures on the number of AIDS cases nationwide, the number of deaths and new cases, and the distribution by age and race, call 404-330-3020; for breakdowns by risk category and sex, call 404-330-3021; for breakdowns by ten leading states and metropolitan areas, call 404-330-3022.

Chlamydia: sexually transmitted disease (STD) causing urethral infection, inflammation of the cervix, pelvic inflammatory disease (PID), and possibly infertility in women.

Chronic: persistent condition of long duration.

Clinical trials: drug trials that use human subjects in an effort to prove drug safety, efficacy, and appropriate dose levels. Clinical trials follow preclinical trials in the test tube and in animals. FDA-mandated trials are divided into phases I, II, and III.

CMV (cytomegalovirus): a virus related to the herpes family. Severe CMV infections can cause opportunistic infections in immunosuppressed individuals. Severe CMV infections can produce hepatitis, pneumonia, retinitis, and colitis, in some cases leading to blindness and chronic diarrhea.

Cofactor: an agent or activity that may increase a person's susceptibility to AIDS. Examples include other infections (besides HIV), drugs, stress, and malnutrition.

Colitis: inflammation of the colon, caused in some cases by CMV.

Compassionate use IND (investigational new drug): informal procedure set up by the FDA permitting use of investigational drugs by individual physicians.

Confidential testing: requires use of your name, which may or may not at some point be made available to the Department of Health, insurance companies, employers, and so on. Reports of people being fired, visited at work, and harassed after their "confidential" test results were disclosed illustrate the risks of abuse of this information and the controversy over this type of testing.

Contact tracing: concept of tracking down all sexual and drug-sharing partners of those with HIV infection, supported by the right wing and some medical groups. The CDC estimates that it would cost up to $7,000 per tracing!

Cunnilingus: oral stimulation of a woman's genitals by tongue and lips.

Contagious: refers to infection communicable by casual contact, such as the common cold or hepatitis A. Neither AIDS nor HIV is contagious; HIV is infectious (communicable only by exchange of blood, semen, and/or vaginal secretions).

Dental dam: 6x6-inch square latex sheet marketed for dentists and dental hygienists that can be used during mouth-to-vagina or mouth-to-anus contact to prevent transmission of HIV or other sexually transmitted diseases.

ELISA (enzyme-linked immunosorbent assay): a blood test that indicates the presence of antibodies to HIV. The ELISA test does not detect HIV itself, but indicates if viral infection has occurred. Increasing incidents of false negatives in women severely call into question this test's efficacy.

Endocarditis: inflammation of the lining of the heart, found mainly in IVDUs as a result of excess bacteria in the blood.

Epidemiology: the study of how diseases are spread.

Epidemic: a disease widespread within a given population; HIV infection is actually a *pandemic,* occurring everywhere and affecting a massive proportion of the population.

False positive: a positive test result for a condition that is in fact negative.

FDA (U.S. Food and Drug Administration): a system of excessive bureaucracy whose responsibility is to approve drugs for testing and treatment. Its decade-long delays, bound in profiteering and red tape, are responsible for the loss of thousands of lives.

Fellatio: stimulation of penis with mouth.

Herpes: family of viruses that include herpes simplex (cold sores), herpes genitalia, CMV, chicken pox, and herpes zoster (shingles). Recurrences of herpes infections are common. Herpes simplex virus-2 (HSV-2) may be considered a cofactor in HIV transmission.

High-risk behavior: a term used to describe activities that increase the risk of transmitting HIV: any activity that allows the blood or semen of one person to contact the blood or mucous membranes of another person, that is, sex without a condom or sharing IV needles. These activities are also referred to as "unsafe" or "unprotected."

HIV (human immunodeficiency virus): a slow-acting virus that is thought to be the sole or foremost causative agent of AIDS.

HIV positive/HIV infected: terms describing a person who has been exposed to and is infected with HIV. Also known as seropositive. This status is determined by a positive lab test for HIV antibodies in the blood.

HIV replication: reproduction of the virus by copying its own RNA onto the DNA of the host, using an enzyme called reverse transcriptase.

HIV spectrum illness: the entire range of medical conditions related to HIV infection and immune system suppression, from asymptomatic seropositivity to AIDS.

HPV: human papillomavirus, associated with genital warts (condyloma) and cervical cancer.

Hyde Amendment: cutoff of federal Medicaid funds for abortion, passed in 1977.

Immune system: the body's system of defense, in which specialized cells and proteins in the blood and other body fluids work together to eliminate disease-producing agents and other toxic foreign substances.

Immunomodulator: a drug that alters, suppresses, or strengthens the immune system.

Immunosuppression: weakening of the immune response that occurs with HIV infection as well as with some antiviral or anticancer treatments.

Informed consent: biomedical or behavioral research and treatment may not be conducted until the legally effective informed consent of each potential subject, or her legally authorized representative, is obtained. Consent forms must explain, in the subject's native language, the purpose and nature of procedures, including foreseeable risks and benefits of participation. Consent must be gained without coercion. Forms must state that consent is voluntary and that at any time the subject may discontinue participation without penalty.

KS (Kaposi's sarcoma): a rare cancer of the connective tissues in blood vessels. Pink or purple blotches on the skin are a symptom of KS. This cancer occurs predominantly among older men and in men with HIV infection; it is rare among women with HIV disease.

Latency period: interval from the time an infectious virus is being reproduced in its host cells to the time symptoms of the infection begin to appear.

MAI (mycobacterium avium intracellulare): pulmonary infection that infects PWAs. It may also affect bone marrow and cause anemia. MAI is often misdiagnosed as the flu.

Mandatory testing: being tested for HIV against your will or without your knowledge.

NIAID (National Institute of Allergy and Infectious Diseases): a branch of the National Institutes of Health, the institute that funds most of the federal government AIDS research and conducts ACTG trials.

Nonoxynol-9 or octoxynol-9: the active ingredient found in most spermicides that inhibits sperm movement and therefore its ability to cause pregnancy and transmit HIV. It should always be used with latex barriers such as dental dams and condoms, but is not effective enough on its own. May cause skin irritation.

Opportunistic infections: infections caused by organisms that do not normally cause infections in people with healthy immune systems, but take advantage of an immune system that is suppressed. The most common opportunistic infections associated with AIDS include PCP, CMV, MAI, and toxoplasmosis. In women, common opportunistic infections are PID, HPV, chronic vaginitis, chlamydia, and endocarditis.

P24 antigen test: test that measures this protein fragment of HIV. A positive result for p24 antigen suggests HIV replication, indicating the virus' level of activity at a specific time.

PCP (pneumocystis carinii pneumonia): common protozoal parasite that multiplies rapidly in the lungs of people who are immunosuppressed. It is the leading cause of death for people with AIDS, but with proper treatment and preventive measures can be controlled.

Pelvic inflammatory disease (PID): general term for an infection that affects a woman's fallopian tubes, ovaries, and/or uterus with widely varying symptoms. Often unnoticed or undiagnosed, PID can develop into various life-threatening conditions.

Placebo: an inert substance against which test drugs are measured. AIDS activists have opposed the use of placebos in drug trials with people who are seriously ill, contending that placebo trials are unethical in life-threatening circumstances.

Prophylaxis: preventive treatment, as aerosolized pentamadine is used for PCP.

Protocol: detailed plan that states a drug trial's rationale, goal, hypothesis, drugs involved, dosage levels, methods of administration, and who may participate, based on their age, sex, and blood levels. All protocols must be approved by an institutions review board (IRB); much precious time is wasted due to poorly designed protocols that are repeatedly sent back to the drawing board.

Retinitis: inflammation of the retina that can be caused by opportunistic infections such as CMV infection.

Retrospective studies: research method that involves looking backward at what has already happened. Includes looking at patient charts or death certificates. It allows for no experimental analysis.

Rimming: stimulation of anus with lips and tongue.

Risk assessment: the act of determining whether you or a (potential) sexual partner have ever been in a situation where exposure to HIV was possible or likely and how that information will affect current or future sexual behavior.

Safe sex: sexual practices that do not transmit HIV.

Safer sex: sexual practices that consider the risk of HIV transmission during a sexual encounter and consider how the risk can be reduced, as in the use of dental dams, condoms, and lubricant containing nonoxynol-9. Safer sex also includes not engaging in an act that doesn't seem safe.

Seroconversion: initial development of antibodies specific to a particular antigen; for example, the development of antibodies to HIV.

Side effect: an unintended effect of a drug, mostly undesirable, harmful, or toxic.

STD (sexually transmitted disease): any disease that can be transmitted or contracted through kissing, sucking, or fucking, otherwise known as "exchange of body fluids." STDs include gonorrhea, syphilis, hepatitis B, chlamydia, herpes, condoloma, chancroid, trichomonas, and others.

Syphilis: STD contracted by kissing, sucking, or fucking; initial infection can be detected by a sore, blister, or chancre on genitals or in mouth, or it can be asymptomatic. Undetected and untreated syphilis can lead to paralysis, dementia, and death.

T-cells: a type of white blood cell (lymphocites) that gives orders to the rest of the immune system. T-cells are the target of HIV. By encoding itself onto their structure, HIV effectively destroys the body's immune system.

T4 (helper)-cells: antibody-triggered immune cells that seek and attack invading organisms. In a healthy immune system there will be twice as many T4-cells as there are T8-cells; in a suppressed immune system the proportion is often reversed.

T4-cell test: test that gives the number and percentage of T4-cells in a blood sample.

T8 (suppressor)-cells: cells in the body that shut down the immune response after it has effectively wiped out invading organisms. While HIV is multiplying, T8-cells are simultaneously attempting to further shut down the immune system, and the percentage of T8-cells often increases in HIV disease.

Toxicity: measure of what quantity of a medicine is poisonous.

Toxoplasmosis: opportunistic protozoal infection affecting the brain.

Vaginitis, chronic: persistent and continuous infection and inflammation in the vagina, often a symptom of HIV infection.

Western Blot: a blood test used to detect antibodies to HIV. It is often used as a secondary confirmation of an initial positive ELISA test because it gives fewer false positive results.

Resources

BEA HANSON

The following list of resources, although not inclusive, represents a range of organizations in various geographical areas that provide AIDS services, treatment, and/or legal assistance for women, as well as teens, lesbians, pregnant women, IVDU/substance users, sex workers, and women in prisons. If materials or services are available in a language other than English, it is indicated at the end of the listing. When contacting HIV-antibody testing services, remember to ask if testing is anonymous (you are identified only by a number) or "confidential" (you must give your name).

For additional resources, call the National AIDS Hotline at 1-800/342-AIDS (1-800/342-2437), or 1-800/344-SIDA (1-800/344-7432) for information in Spanish. The TDY number is 1-800/243-7889 (English only). You can call the hotline toll-free, 24 hours a day, seven days a week. The hotline maintains a computerized list of names and phone numbers for organizations across the country, including HIV counseling and testing centers, drug treatment services, general AIDS information, hotlines in each state, and teen and runaway services.

General Resources

Northeastern States

AIDS Action Committee
140 Clarendon Street, Boston, MA 02116
617/437-6200
    Counseling, support groups, meals, transportation, and financial and rental assistance

AIDS Coalition to Unleash Power (ACT UP)
496 Hudson Street, Suite 4G, New York, NY 10014
212/989-1114
    AIDS activist organization

The AIDS Project
22 Monument Square, 5th floor, Portland, ME 04101
207/774-6877
Support groups, hotline, HIV testing and counseling, financial assistance, and meals program

AIDS Project at the Women's Clinic
Community Family Planning Council
910 E. 172nd Street, Bronx, NY 10454
212/991-9250
HIV testing and counseling, support groups, street outreach, and education (Spanish)

AIDS Project New Haven
P.O. Box 636, New Haven, CT 06503
203/624-0947
Buddy program, case management services, massage clinic, interfaith network, meal delivery, support groups, counseling, hotline, and education

American Foundation for AIDS Research (AmFAR)
1515 Broadway, Suite 3601, New York, NY 10036
212/719-0033
Education, information, and referral

Amigas Latinas en Acción Pro-Salud
47 Nichols Avenue, Watertown, MA 02172
617/491-1268
Education, counseling, and referral (Spanish)

Black Women's Health Council
P.O. Box 4331, Upper Marlboro, MD 20775
301/322-4707
Training program for service providers in low-income areas, and support groups for teens

Blacks Educating Blacks About Sexual Health Issues (BEBASHI)
1528 Walnut Street, Philadelphia, PA 19102
215/546-4140
Sexuality workshops and AIDS education

Body Positive
208 West 13th Street, New York, NY 10011
212/633-1782
Counseling, support, and monthly holistic/alternative newsletter

Boston Women's AIDS Information Project
c/o Fenway Community Health Center
16 Haviland Street, Boston, MA 02115
617/267-0900
Community-based training and education for women of color

Brooklyn AIDS Task Force—Women's Initiative
22 Chapel Street, Brooklyn, NY 11201
718/638-AIDS
Free AIDS information and support groups (Spanish)

Chinatown Health Clinic - AIDS Project
Health Education Dept., 89 Baxter Street, New York, NY 10013
212/732-9547
Education workshops, videos, and pamphlets in Chinese

Family Health Project
17 Murray Street, New York, NY 10007
212/749-6957
Information, education, meal programs, and support for women and their families

Gay Men's Health Crisis
129 West 20th Street, New York, NY 10011
212/807-6655
Confidential information for all PWAs, including counseling, legal services, housing referral, social events, and educational materials (Spanish and Creole)

Haitian Coalition on AIDS
50 Court Street, Room 605, Brooklyn, NY 11201
718/855-7275
Education (Creole)

Haitian Women's Program/AFSC
15 Rutherford Place, New York, NY 10003
212/598-0965
Community workshops and trainings for health care workers (Creole)

Health Education Resource Organization (HERO)
101 West Read Street, Suite 822, Baltimore, MD 21201
301/685-1180 and 301/945-AIDS (hotline)
Counseling, support groups, legal assistance, advocacy, buddy program, financial assistance, and referral

Hispanic AIDS Forum
121 Avenue of the Americas, Suite 505, New York, NY 10013
212/966-6336
Education, advocacy, HIV testing information, counseling, hotline, and referral

Hyacinth Foundation/New Jersey AIDS Project
211 Livingston Avenue, New Brunswick, NJ 08901
201/246-0204 or 1-800/433-0254
Counseling, including PWAs in prison

The Jose Gonzalez House
1177 Hoe Avenue, Bronx, NY 10459
212/378-3313
Transitional facility for homeless PWAs, with case management,

advocacy, and referral

Lower East Side Women's Center
P.O. Box 1776, Peter Stuyvesant Station, New York, NY 10009
212/353-1924
Referral services

Minority Task Force on AIDS - Women's Action Committee
92 St. Nicholas Avenue, New York, NY 10030
212/749-2816
Counseling, buddy program, benefits assistance, support groups, hotline, publications, outreach, and education

People With AIDS Coalition
31 West 26th Street, New York, NY 10010
212/532-0290
Support groups, referral, and monthly newsletter

Sister-To-Sister Project
718/596-6000
Support groups of Black women coping with HIV infection

Women and AIDS Resource Network (WARN)
P.O. Box 020525, Brooklyn, NY 11202
718/596-6007
Counseling, referrals, workshops for women PWAs

Women in Crisis - Minority Women and AIDS Project
c/o Project Return Foundation
133 West 21st Street, New York, NY 10011
212/242-4880
Street outreach

Women In Need - AIDS Project
406 West 40th Street, New York, NY 10018
212/695-7330
Education, outreach in shelters and transitional housing, support groups, and day care for children of homeless women

Women's Action Alliance
370 Lexington Avenue, New York, NY 10017
212/532-8330
Resource guides and educational materials

Women's Institute for Training and Support Services
204 West 20th Street, New York, NY 10011
212/924-8402
Support groups, meditation classes, nutritional counseling, and natural detoxification for women

Women's Network, AIDS Education Project
2127 Third Avenue, New York, NY 10035
212/369-4211
Education and support groups

Southeastern States
AIDS Atlanta
1132 West Peachtree NW, Atlanta, GA 30309-3624
404/872-0600 and 404/876-9944 (AIDS Infoline)
Counseling, street outreach, education, and referral

AIDS Services of Austin
P.O. Box 4874, Austin, TX 78765
512/472-2273 and 512/472-2001 (Spanish)
Counseling, advocacy, educational materials, and referral

Alianza
P.O. Box 53396, Washington, DC 20009
202/223-9600
Education, support groups, counseling, and referral (Spanish)

Health Crisis Network
1351 NW 20th Street, Miami, FL 33142
305/326-8833
Referral, counseling, and support groups (Spanish and Creole)

National AIDS Network
2033 M Street, NW, 18th floor, Washington, DC 20036
202/293-2437
Nationwide resource center and clearinghouse

National Association of People With AIDS
2025 I Street, NW, Washington, DC 20006
202/429-2856
Self-empowerment of People with AIDS/ARC through education and support

National Black Women's Health Project
1237 Gordon Street, SW, Atlanta, GA 30310
404/753-0916
Self-help support groups, health advocacy, and education

National Women's Health Network
1325 G Street, NW, Washington, DC 20005
202/347-1140
Clearinghouse, education, and referral

NO/AIDS Task Force
P.O. Box 2616, New Orleans, LA 70126
504/891-3732
Counseling, educational information, and referral

North Carolina AIDS Control Program
P.O. Box 27687, Raleigh, NC 27611
919/733-7301
HIV testing and counseling, buddy programs, support groups, educational materials, and referrals

North Central Florida AIDS Network
1124 NW 39th Avenue, Suite B, Gainesville, FL 32605
904/372-4370
    Support groups, pre- and post-HIV test counseling, buddy program, and educational materials

Sisterlove Women's AIDS Project
1132 W. Peachtree Street, Atlanta, GA 30309
404/872-0600
    Safe-sex information, workshops, advocacy for women with AIDS, with an emphasis on serving women of color

South Carolina AIDS Education Network
c/o MDM Enterprises
2768 Decker Boulevard, Suite 98, Columbia, SC 29206
    Drop-in AIDS education center for women and children, including videos, safe-sex kits (for sale), and teen AIDS drama club (all run out of a beauty parlor)

Women's Council on AIDS
1441 Florida Avenue, NW, Washington, DC 20009
202/387-4898
    Support groups, outreach, education, safe-sex education parties, hospital outreach, and training

Midwestern States

Aliveness Project
730 East 38th Street, Minneapolis, MN 55407
612/822-7946
    Women's support group, meals, drop-in center, clothing, library, massage therapy, acupuncture, chiropractics

Community Health Awareness Group
3028 East Grand Boulevard, Detroit, MI 48202
313/872-2424
    Community-based program for African-American and Latin communities, including counseling, support groups, HIV and TB testing, referrals, bleach distribution, home visits, food, and clothing.

Indian Health Board of Minneapolis
1315 East 24th Street, Minneapolis, MN 55404
612/721-7425
    Case management, peer youth teams, support groups, spiritual advisement, and education

Kupona Network - Women's Project
4611 South Ellis, Chicago, IL 60653
312/536-3000
    Education, prevention, safe-sex workshops, counseling, case management, support groups, advocacy, and referral

Minnesota American Indian AIDS Task Force
1433 East Franklin Avenue, Minneapolis, MN 55404
612/870-1723
Technical assistance, workshops, resource development, outreach, educational materials, and video

Native American Women's Health Education Resource Center
P.O. Box 572, Lake Andes, SD 57356
605/487-7072
First reservation-based women's health resource center; culturally specific health education, child development, domestic abuse, and advocacy program

Simon House
16260 Dexter Avenue, Detroit, MI 48221
313/863-1400
Transitional house for women with AIDS and their children; hospice, parenting and nutrition classes, referrals, advocacy

St. Louis Efforts for AIDS
4050 Lindell Boulevard, St. Louis, MO 63108
314/531-2847
Support groups, buddy program, counseling, referrals, and educational materials

Topeka AIDS Project
P.O. Box 4726, Topeka, KS 66604
913/232-3100
Only direct care agency for PWAs in the area; support groups, buddy program, home health care, child care, and education

Wellness Networks, Inc.
P.O. Box 1046, Royal Oak, MI 48068
313/547-9040 and 800/872-2437 (inside Michigan only)
Support groups and buddy system; local chapters in eight other Michigan cities

Western States

Asian AIDS Project
300 Fourth Street, Suite 3401, San Francisco, CA 94107
415/227-0946
Education/prevention in Chinese dialects, Japanese, Vietnamese, Korean, and others

Black Coalition on AIDS
333 Valencia Street, Room 101, San Francisco, CA 94112
415/553-8197
Advocacy, training, workshops, and outreach to the Black community

Cascade AIDS Project
408 S.W. Second Avenue, Room 412, Portland, OR 97204
503/223-5907
Support groups, alcohol and drug recovery, counseling, educational materials, community health nurse, free legal advice, emergency financial aid, and hotline

Colorado AIDS Project
1576 Sherman, Denver, CO 80203
303/837-0166 or 1-800/333-2437 (outside Denver)
Counseling, information, referral, emergency financial assistance, buddy program, and support groups

Latino AIDS Project
2401 24th Street, San Franicsco, CA 94110
415/647-5450
Mental health clinic, entitlements benefits, advocacy, counseling, and support groups (in Spanish)

Minority AIDS Project
5149 West Jefferson Boulevard, Los Angeles, CA 90016
213/936-4949
Street outreach, support groups, food, clothing, financial assistance, and counseling (Spanish)

Multicultural Alliance for the Prevention of AIDS (MAPA)
1625 Carroll Street, San Francisco, CA 94124
415/822-7500
Advocacy, outreach, food and clothing bank

National Native American AIDS Prevention Center
6239 College Avenue, #201, Oakland, CA 94618
415/658-2051
Information and training for Native American communities

Native American AIDS Advisory Board of California
2020 Hurley Avenue, Suite 155, Sacramento, CA 95825
916/929-9761
Advocacy, counseling, training, and health education materials

People of Color Against AIDS Network
1200 S. Jackson, Suite 25 & 26, Seattle, WA 98144
206/322-7061
Prevention, outreach, and educational materials

Project AWARE
Ward 84, San Francisco General Hospital
995 Potrero Avenue, San Francisco, CA 94110
415/376-4091
AIDS research and health promotion for heterosexual women

San Francisco AIDS Foundation
333 Valencia Street, 4th floor, San Francisco, CA 94103
415/864-4376 or 800/863-AIDS (hotline)
Social services, food bank, emergency housing, and education programs and materials

Women and AIDS Risk Network Project L.A.
900 N. Alvarado, 2nd floor, Los Angeles, CA 90026
213/413-7779
Counseling, court referral for sex workers, support groups, and outreach

Women's AIDS Network
333 Valencia Street, 4th floor, San Francisco, CA 94103
415/864-4589

Treatment Resources

AIDS Project Los Angeles
6721 Romaine Street, Los Angeles, CA 90038
213/962-1600
Hotlines: 213/876-AIDS (in L.A.) 800/922-AIDS (in S. CA)
            800/222-SIDA (in Spanish) 800/553-AIDS (TTY)
Counseling, support groups, insurance counseling, dental and mental health care, and free food, clothing, and medical assistance for those who meet criteria

AIDS Treatment Registry
P.O. Box 30234, New York, NY 10011-0102
212/268-4196
Information, educational materials, and access to AIDS-related clinical drug trials

Community Health Project
208 West 13th Street, New York, NY 10011
212/675-3559
Outpatient medical care, support groups, counseling, education, and referral

Community Research Initiative
155 West 23rd Street, New York, NY 10011
212/481-1050
Community-based research organization developing clinical trials for experimental AIDS treatment

Fenway Community Health Center
16 Haviland Street, Boston, MA 02115
617/267-0900
Outpatient medical care, gynecological services, substance use treatment and counseling including acupuncture detox, counseling, nutrition information, massage, holistic therapy, and HIV testing

Health Education AIDS Liaison (HEAL)
P.O. Box 1103, Old Chelsea Station, New York, NY 10011
212/674-4673
Alternative and holistic approaches

Howard Brown Memorial Clinic
945 West George Street, Chicago, IL 60657
312/871-5777
Medical services, HIV testing and counseling, support groups, massage therapy, education, and training

Innovative Community Enterprises (ICE), The AIDS Co-op
P.O. Box 1061, Cooper Station, New York, NY 10276
212/529-8200
Affordable prices for AIDS treatment drugs in New York area

New York State AIDS Drug Assistance Program (ADAP)
800/542-AIDS
Subsidized AIDS-related drug program

Northern Lights Alternatives
78 West 75th Street, New York, NY 10023
212/337-8747 or 877-4846
Holistic support

Project Inform
347 Dolores Street, San Francisco, CA 94110
800/822-7422
Nationwide referral to treatment centers and treatment information

Sable/Scherer Clinic of Cook County Hospital
1835 West Harrison, Chicago, IL 60612
312/633-5182
Free confidential medical services, pre- and post-test counseling, and a women's clinic (Spanish)

Shiprock Community Health Center
P.O. Box 1734, Shiprock, NM 87420
505/368-5181
Outreach, HIV testing and counseling, gynecological services, support groups, workshops, and referrals for Native American communities

St. Marks Women's Health Collective
9 Second Avenue, New York, NY 10003
212/228-7482
Gynecological exams, AIDS counseling, and HIV testing

Whitman-Walker Clinic, Women's Committee on AIDS
2335 18th Street, NW, Washington, DC 20009
202/797-3500
Medical services, HIV testing and counseling, support groups, legal assistance, housing referrals, and education

The Women's AIDS Project
8235 Santa Monica Boulevard, Suite 201, West Hollywood, CA 90046
213/650-1508
    Support groups, HIV testing and counseling, gynecological services, workshops, and education

Resources for Teens

Adolescent AIDS Program, Montefiore Medical Center
111 East 210th Street, Bronx, NY 10467
212/920-2179
    Medical evaluation and HIV testing and counseling

Adolescent Treatment and Education Alliance
2751 Mary Street, La Crescenta, CA 91214
818/248-2623
    Education services and peer education training

The DOOR
127 6th Avenue, New York, NY 10013
212/941-9090
    Counseling, HIV testing, and educational materials for runaway and homeless youth

Mount Sinai Hospital Adolescent Health Center
Box 1005, New York, NY 10029
212/241-TEEN
    Medical services, birth control information and materials, and counseling

Neon Street
3227 North Sheffield, Chicago, IL 60657
312/528-7767
    Support and counseling services, and sexuality and health education for homeless teens

Teens and AIDS Hotline
800/234-TEEN
    Nationwide referral service

Legal Resources

AIDS Law Project, Gay and Lesbian Advocates and Defenders
P.O. Box 218, Boston, MA 02112
617/426-1350
    Counseling, class-action lawsuits, and education

American Bar Association Immigration Law Project
1800 M Street, NW, Washington, DC 20036
202/331-2268
    Educational materials for advocates and attorneys on discrimination against HIV-positive immigrants

American Civil Liberties Union AIDS Project
132 West 43rd Street, New York, NY 10036
212/944-9800, ext. 545
   Litigation and educational materials

Coalition for Immigrant and Refugee Rights
301 Mission Street, Suite 400, San Francisco, CA 94105
415/543-9444
   Legislative advocacy, litigation, and information for HIV-positive people applying for amnesty

Lambda Legal Defense and Education Fund
666 Broadway, New York, NY 10012
212/995-8585
   Litigation and educational projects for lesbian and gay legal rights

National Lawyers Guild AIDS Network
588 Capp Street, San Francisco, CA 94102
415/824-8884
   Advocacy, litigation, and referral

Resources for Lesbians

Gay and Lesbian Adolescent Social Services (GLASS)
8235 Santa Monica Boulevard #214, West Hollywood, CA 90046
213/656-5005
   Counseling, education, housing, and medical referrals

Hetrick-Martin Institute
401 West Street, New York, NY 10014
212/633-8920 and 212/633-8926 (TTY)
   Counseling, support groups, and social activities for lesbian and gay youth

National Gay and Lesbian Task Force
1517 U Street, NW, Washington, DC 20009
202/332-6483
   Activism, lobbying, advocacy, and referral

National Lesbian and Gay Crisis Line
800/SOS-GAYS
   Counseling, education, and referral

National Lesbian and Gay Health Foundation
1638 R Street, NW, #2, Washington, DC 20009
202/797-3708
   Health care advocacy, clearinghouse, publishes annual directory of lesbian/gay health services

Resources for Pregnant Women

Manhattan Teen Pregnancy Network
285 West Broadway, Room 320, New York, NY 10013
212/219-8835
Outreach to high school teens, information, and referral

Pediatric and Pregnancy AIDS Hotline
Albert Einstein College of Medicine
1300 Morris Park Avenue, Bronx, NY 10461
212/430-3333
Counseling, information, and referral

Resources for Intravenous Drug Users/Substance Users

Association for Drug Abuse Prevention and Treatment (ADAPT)
236 East 111th Street, New York, NY 10029
212/289-1957
Street outreach, advocacy, and counseling

Chemical Dependency Center for Women
1507 21st Street, Suite 100, Sacramento, CA 95814
916/448-2951
Counseling, street and prison outreach, and education

Health Crisis Network
P.O. Box 42-1280, Miami, FL 33242-1280
305/634-4636
Individual and group counseling for substance users

Mid-City Consortium on AIDS
1779 Haight Street, San Francisco, CA 94117
415/751-4221
Street-based AIDS education/prevention project for IV drug users

Promesa
1776 Clay Avenue, Bronx, NY 10453
212/299-1100
Counseling, in- and outpatient methadone and drug-free detoxification
programs (Spanish)

Resources for Sex Workers

California Prostitutes Education Project (CAL-PEP)
333 Valencia Street #213, San Francisco, CA 94103
415/558-0450
Advocacy, support groups, buddy program, HIV testing and counseling,
education, outreach, prevention, and referral

COYOTE/National Task Force on Prostitution
333 Valencia Street, #213, San Francisco, CA 94103
415/558-0450
Lobbying for prostitutes' rights and umbrella organization for local prostitute advocacy and activist organizations

Genesis House
911 West Addison, Chicago, IL 60613
312/281-3917
Lock-up presentations, street outreach, and educational materials

Hooking is Real Employment (HIRE)
404/876-1212
Support groups, advocacy, legal referrals, and educational materials for women in the sex industry

L.A. COYOTE
1626 North Wilcox, #580, Hollywood, CA 90028
213/389-4495
Prodecriminalization organization providing counseling for arrested prostitutes, legal referrals, and public education

Pink Ladies Social Club
12439 Magnolia Blvd., Suite 218, N. Hollywood, CA 91607
Porn-star support group and newsletter for women in adult video industry

Prostitutes of New York and Friends (PONY)
c/o P.O. Box 1331, Old Chelsea Station, New York, NY 10011
212/713-5678
Prodecriminalization organization, political and support groups, health committee, newsletter, and safer-sex information

US PROStitutes Collective (US PROS)
P.O. Box 14512, San Francisco, CA 94114
415/558-9628
Direct action, legal referral, and AIDS education materials advocating abolition of all prostitute laws

Resources for Women in Prisons

AIDS Counseling and Education (ACE)
Bedford Hills Correctional Facility
287 Harris Road, Bedford Hills, New York 10507
914/241-3100, ext. 260
Peer counseling and education group among prisoners; inmate and worker education, workshops for general public, and nationwide model for peer education for other prisons

National Prison Project
1616 P Street, NW, Washington, DC 20036
202/331-0500
Information, studies, and referrals

Bibliography

POLLY THISTLETHWAITE

Alexander, Priscilla, *Prostitutes Prevent AIDS: A Manual for Health Educators,* California Prostitutes Education Project (CAL-PEP, P.O. Box 6297, San Francisco, CA 94101-6297), 1988.

Formed by the prostitutes' rights organization COYOTE, CAL-PEP exists to educate sex workers, and their clients and other sex partners, about HIV and AIDS. This handbook outlines a training program designed to do that; also emphasizes the need to eradicate the insane police practice of confiscating condoms, spermicides, bleach bottles, and drug paraphernalia during arrests. Appendices include safer-sex and drug-use guidelines, organizations of prostitutes in the United States, prostitution laws and enforcement practices, and studies of HIV infection among North American prostitutes.

Alonso, Ana Maria and Maria Teresa Koreck, "Silences: 'Hispanics,' AIDS, and Sexual Practices," *Differences,* Vol. 1:1, Winter 1989.

"In order for AIDS research to advance, the category 'Hispanic' needs to be dismantled," explain the authors, as do the culture-laden constructions of sexuality.

Alternative Press Index: An Index to Alternative and Radical Publications, Baltimore: Alternative Press Center, July/December 1969-.

API was founded by radical librarians right after Stonewall. It currently indexes over 230 queer, feminist, and radical publications nobody else will, including: *The Advocate, Black/Out, Covert Action, Fag Rag, Gay Community News, Lesbian Contradiction, Mother Jones, The Nation, off our backs, Rites, Spare Rib, Trivia,* and *Zeta Magazine. API* and *Women Studies Abstracts* are essential for finding information on women, AIDS, and activism in the queer and radical press.

American College Health Association, *Women & AIDS,* Rockville, MD: ACHA (15879 Crabbs Branch Way, Rockville, MD 20855), 1988.

Best brochure we've seen on safer sex for women. It includes a section about dental dams.

"Antibody to Human Immunodeficiency Virus in Female Prostitutes," *Morbidity and Mortality Weekly Report,* Vol. 36:11, March 27, 1987.

Reprinted in the April 17, 1987 *Journal of the American Medical Association,* this oft-cited report combines data from seven wildly varying studies of U.S. women. Analysis is biased, thin, and faulty.

Barker-Benfield, G. J., *The Horrors of the Half-Known Life: Male Attitudes Toward Women and Sexuality in Nineteenth-Century America*, New York: Harper & Row, 1976.

An in-depth examination of men's thoughts about women and the rise of western gynecology.

Black/Out: The Magazine of the National Coalition for Black Lesbians and Gays, Detroit: NCBLG (19641 West Seven Mile, Detroit, MI 48219), Vol. 2:1, Fall 1988.

This issue commemorates the 10th anniversary of NCBLG. There are several pieces about AIDS, including contributions on women of color and AIDS by Lynell Johnson and Ayofemi Stowe. *Black/Out* is published in May and October.

The Body Positive: A Magazine About HIV, New York: Body Positive (2095 Broadway, Suite 306, New York, NY 10023, 212/721-1619), October 1987-.

This free monthly magazine contains articles on current issues in HIV treatment and politics. Also contains extensive resource listings, including those specifically for women. Important articles about women and HIV include Alice Terson's "All About Alice," November 1989; Denise Ribble's "Barriers to Health Care for Women with HIV," July/August 1989; and "Children and HIV," February 1990. Body Positive is a wonderful, multifaceted support organization of and for seropositive people.

Bohne, John, Tom Cunningham, Jon Engbretson, Ken Fornataro, and Mark Harrington, *Treatment and Data Handbook: Treatment Designs*, New York: ACT UP, 1989.

This is an unpublished document, but you still might be able to get one if you call or write.

Boston Women's Health Book Collective, *The New Our Bodies, Ourselves: a Book By and For Women*, New York: Simon & Schuster, 1984.

First issued in 1972, this is a classic radical resource on feminist health practice. Geared mainly for straight, able-bodied women, it includes some work on lesbian sexuality and relationships. Not much in here about AIDS, though there is a section on STDs.

Brandt, Alan, "The Syphilis Epidemic and Its Relation to AIDS," *Science*, January 1988.

—, *No Magic Bullet: A Social History of Venereal Disease in the United States Since 1880*, New York: Oxford University Press, 1985.

The history of the social and political (mal)treatment of STDs is an ugly one. Brandt's analyses speak as much to our modern HIV epidemic as it does to past treatment of VD. The histories of public health policy, sex education, and prostitution point to a legacy of ineffective government action taken at the expense of oppressed people. Also see "A Historical Perspective" in Dalton and Burris annotated below.

Bridgham, Bethany J., ed., *A Summary of AIDS Laws From the 1988 Legislative Sessions*, Washington, D.C.: George Washington University, Intergovernmental Health Policy Project (2011 I St., N.W., Suite 200, Washington, D.C. 20006, 202/872-1445), April 1989.

A summary of state laws running the gamut of HIV issues: testing, bathhouses, partner notification, discrimination, pregnant women. This is for legal documentation only; there's no analysis.

Bristow, Ann, Andrea Devine, and Denise McWilliams, "AIDS and Women in Prison," *Gay Community News*, August 27 - September 5, 1987.

A good primer, though lots has happened since 1987.

Byron, Peg, "Women With AIDS—Untold Stories," Village Voice, September 24, 1985.

This was the first feature in the *Voice* about women and AIDS. Byron has also written about activism, sexuality, and lesbian and gay health concerns for a number of publications, like *Womanews* and *Gay Community News*.

Califia, Pat, *Sapphistry: The Book of Lesbian Sexuality*, Tallahassee, FL: Naiad Press, 1988.

Explicit talk about queer girl sex, and how to do it safer. Califia includes "A Note on Lesbians and AIDS" that talks about how to use gloves, condoms, dams, toys, and other gear. Also tells you how to clean your works. Wouldn't it be smart for more porn and sex publications to include basic safe-sex information? For safer sex from top to bottom, see *The Lesbian S/M Safety Manual: Basic Health and Safety for Woman-to-Woman S/M* (Denver: Lace Publications, 1988), which Califia edited. And if you like that, you'll love *Macho Sluts* (Alyson Publications, 1988) for more erotic/safer-sex fiction. Dykes can watch out for more safe-sex info and erotica in lesbo porn and politic rags *Bad Attitude* and *On Our Backs*.

Cameron, D.W., et al., "Female to Male Transmission of Human Immunodeficiency Virus Type 1: Risk Factors for Seroconversion in Men," *Lancet*, Vol. 8860, No. 2, 1989.

This study conducted in Nairobi indicates genital ulcers on penises are a heavy factor in female-to-male transmission.

Carlomusto, Jean, "Deep Inside Safer Sex Videos," *On Our Backs*, January/February 1990.

The inside story of making the lesbo safer-sex porn video *Current Flow*.

Carter, Erica and Simon Watney, eds., *Taking Liberties: AIDS and Cultural Politics*, London: Serpent's Tail, 1989.

This collection "emerges" from the papers read at the March 1988 London conference at the Institute of Contemporary Arts (ICA). Contains 15 pieces, including Lynne Segal's "Lessons From the Past: Feminism, Sexual Politics and the Challenge of AIDS," and Watney's "AIDS, Language and the Third World."

Chiaramonte, Lee, "Lesbian Safety and AIDS: The Very Last Fairy Tale," *Visibilities*, January/February 1988.

Chiaramonte discusses the ins and outs of lesbian sexual transmission, invisibility, and epidemiology. *Visibilities* (Box 1258 Stuyvesant Station, New York, NY 10009) is a bimonthly publication since 1987, with a regular column now on women and AIDS/HIV.

Chirimuuta, Richard and Rosalind Chirimuuta, *AIDS, Africa and Racism*, Derbyshire: UK (Bretby House, Stanhope, Bretby, Nr. Burton-on-Trent, Derbyshire, DE15 OPT, UK), 1987.

Challenges the Panos Institute's statistics for AIDS cases in Central Africa by pointing out the high false positivity rate of testing there. Questions the motives of the European sponsors of this study, charging the Panos Institute with ignorance of African government structures and operations.

Clarke, Loren and Malcolm Potts, eds., *The AIDS Reader: A Documentary History of a Modern Epidemic*, Boston: Branden Publishing Co., 1988.

Reprints some stuff of interest including Jane Gross' *New York Times* article,

"The Bleak and Lonely Lives of Women Who Carry AIDS."

Committee for Abortion Rights and Against Sterilization Abuse (CARASA), Susan Davis, ed., *Woman Under Attack: Victories, Backlash, and the Fight for Reproductive Freedom*, Boston: South End Press, 1988.

CARASA first published this pamphlet in 1979. The group developed the politics of reproductive freedom, which expands the politics of reproductive rights, striving for "freedom from" legal interventions, to call for the transformation of social conditions which would allow us real "freedom to" make choices about our lives.

Corea, Gena, *The Hidden Malpractice: How American Medicine Mistreats Women*, New York: Harper & Row, 1985.

First published in 1977, Part One of this book deals with women being "barred from healing." The second part addresses the detrimental impact this has on the health care women receive.

Crimp, Douglas, ed., *AIDS: Cultural Analysis/Cultural Activism*, Cambridge, MA: MIT Press, 1988.

An important, intelligent anthology reflecting a range of AIDS activist sensibilities. Chapters devoted to women's issues include Suki Ports' "Needed (For Women and Children)" and Carol (COYOTE) Leigh's "Further Violations of Our Rights." Other contributions (one by the PWA Coalition, for example) speak to women's specific needs for AIDS education and health care.

Dalton, Harlon, Scott Burris, and the Yale Law AIDS Project, eds., *AIDS and the Law*, New Haven, CT: Yale University Press, 1987.

Contains legal information and analysis, including John F. Decker's piece on aspects of prostitution, regulation, testing, and the like.

Davis, Angela, *Women, Culture, & Politics*, New York: Random House, 1989.
—, *Women, Race & Class*, New York: Random House, 1981.

Davis traces political solidarity and antagonism in terms of class, race, and sex in U.S. women's history. *Women, Race & Class* includes the chapter "Racism, Birth Control, and Reproductive Rights," which speaks to the politics around women and HIV/AIDS as well. *Women, Culture, & Politics* includes more recent lectures and writings. See especially her chapter on the politics of Black women's health, with description and discussion of the National Black Women's Health Project.

Delacoste, Frederique and Priscilla Alexander, eds., *Sex Work: Writings by Women in the Sex Industry*, Pittsburgh: Cleis Press, 1987.

Sex workers tell it well in this anthology of essays, prose, and poetry. All voices unite in speaking cogently to the struggle to end violence against prostitutes. Includes articles on U.S. and European sex worker organizations, among them WHISPER, COYOTE/NTPR, ICPR, U.S. PROS, The Red Thread/Pink Thread.

Directory of Clinical Trials and Experimental AIDS/HIV Treatments in New York and New Jersey, AIDS Treatment Registry, Inc., P.O. Box 30234, New York, NY 10011-0102. 212/268-4196. Bimonthly, free/donation.

ATR is a community-based organization that informs and advocates for women, men, and children involved in clinical drug trials. The *Directory* serves as a primary outlet for information about new drugs and trials, indicating if women are excluded from trials or not. ATR also distributes educational material and conducts seminars for trial participants. With experimental drugs being a predominant treatment for HIV-related illness, this information is vital.

Dobie, Kathy, "The Invisible Girls: Homeless and Hooking in the Neighborhood," *Village Voice*, March 14, 1990.

A story about the so-called "new prostitution" fed by crack addiction. Dobie met women interviewed for this article through ADAPT's Yolanda Serrano. Daniel Lazare's "Crack and AIDS: The Next Wave?" *Village Voice*, May 8, 1990, is a hip little piece about the relationship between crack, sex, and HIV transmission.

—, "Yolanda Serrano," *Ms.*, January/February 1989.

Profiles the director of Association for Drug Abuse Prevention and Treatment (ADAPT), one of *Ms.*' six women of the year.

Ehrenreich, Barbara, *American Health Empire: Power, Profits, and Politics*, New York: Random House, 1970.

Classic account of the transformation of the medical establishment from community-based cottage industry to the modern alienated empire.

—and Dierdre English, *Complaints and Disorders: the Sexual Politics of Sickness*, New York: The Feminist Press, 1973.

Discusses the role of medicine and women in 19th century class struggle. Also see their *For Her Own Good: 150 Years of the Experts' Advice to Women*, Garden City, NY: Anchor, 1979, for analysis of the role of male scientific, uh, "expertise" in exerting control over women. Ehrenreich and English's *Witches, Midwives, and Healers*, New York: Feminist Press, 1973, examines medieval religious witch hunts as persecution of women's sexuality for patriarchal gain. Parallels abound.

Einhorn, Lena, "New Data on Lesbians and AIDS," *off our backs*, April 1989.

The CDC later cleaned up the 164 reported cases of AIDS among lesbian and bisexual women; polished it down to a shiny 100.

Elze, Diane, interviewer, "Underground Abortion: Memories of Chicago's Jane Collective," *Sojourner*, April/May and June/July 1988.

Jane ruled Chicago before Roe, and we'll do it again if we have to. See this wonderful two-part interview with Janes 1, 2, and 3 for details. Also see "Just Call 'Jane'," a first-person account by a Jane Collective member, published in *From Abortion to Reproductive Freedom*, ed., Marlene Gerber Fried, Boston: South End Press, 1990; and also, Pauline Bart's "Seizing the Means of Reproduction: An Illegal Feminist Abortion Collective—How and Why it Worked," available from The Boston Women's Health Book Collective in Somerville, MA.

The Facts About AIDS, HIV, and You, New York: Hetrick-Martin Institute, 1989.

An excellent pamphlet for gay, lesbian, and heterosexual teens about HIV basics. Check it out: "Abstaining from sexual intercourse is one way to protect yourself from HIV. But you don't have to give up or avoid sex..." And it goes on to specify. *Lynda Madras Talks to Teens about AIDS*, New York: New Market Press, 1988, is more widely available in bookstores. It's OK, but not particularly sex positive for teens.

Federation of Feminist Women's Health Centers, *A New View of a Woman's Body*, New York: Simon and Schuster, 1981.

With excellent graphics and drawings by Suzann Gage, this is a lovely textual guide to female bodies. Also see the Federation's *How to Stay Out of the Gynecologist's Office*, Culver City, CA: Peace Press, 1981.

Fee, Elizabeth and Daniel Fox, eds., *AIDS: The Burdens of History,* Berkeley, CA: University of California Press, 1988.

Includes Paula Treichler's straight feminist academic construct "AIDS, Gender, and Biomedical Discourse: Current Contests for Meaning," which is interesting if you have the inclination to wade through the jargon.

V International Conference on AIDS: The Scientific and Social Challenge. Abstracts. Ottawa, Canada: International Development Research Centre, 1989.

This is the 7-lb. conference program that briefly summarizes most of the papers presented at the conference. There are 5,539 entries in total; a few are mentioned in this book. Some of the papers have been published, others haven't. Like other conference programs and proceedings, this tome is not widely available, unfortunately. Papers from the first conference have only recently been marketed, see Fleming, Alan, et al., eds., *The Global Impact of AIDS: Proceedings of the I International Conference on the Global Impact of AIDS,* New York: Liss, 1988.

Fumento, Michael, *The Myth of Heterosexual AIDS: How a Tragedy Has Been Distorted by the Media and Partisan Politics,* New York: Basic Books, 1990.

This book is full of heterosexist, sexist bullshit. It is as malicious as Dr. Robert Gould's January 1988 article in *Cosmo,* and James Petersen's "Unrealistic Fear" in *Playboy,* July 1988.

Gage, Suzann, *When Birth Control Fails: How to Abort Ourselves Safely,* Hollywood: Speculum Press, 1979.

Yep, a do-it-yourself guide. It's not that we couldn't do it regularly if the skills and instruction weren't so privileged. A real prospect to ponder as *Roe v. Wade* falls. Also see Jane Post-Webster's (get it? post-*Webster...*) "Sisters Doing It For Themselves," *Outweek,* September 24, 1989.

Gay Community News, 62 Berkeley Street, Boston, MA 02116. Weekly. 1973-.

The queer activist community paper of record, just witness all the cites in this bibliography alone. Read *GCN* for smart coverage of national issues, with a slant toward Boston, of course.

Gay Men's Health Crisis, *Legal Answers About AIDS,* GMHC (Box 274, 132 W. 24th St., New York, NY 10011, 212/807-6655), 1988.

A concise pocket-sized legal guide for PWAs prepared by Mark Senak. GMHC has other free pamphlets, but most aren't geared for women. Also see GMHC's *Women Need to Know About AIDS* (1988). *The Safer Sex Condom Guide* (1987) is for men and women. It's got pictures...of penises.

Giddings, Paula, *When and Where I Enter: The Impact of Black Women on Race and Sex in America.* New York: William Morrow, 1984.

A narrative history of Black women activists in the United States outlining personal and institutional confrontations with racism and sexism. This will enrich your understanding of the struggle and how HIV affects women's lives.

Gostin, Larry O., "Public Health Strategies for Confronting AIDS: Legislative and Regulatory Policy in the United States," *Journal of the American Medical Association,* Vol. 261:11, March 17, 1989.

Discusses the legal specifics of a range of government strategies including HIV testing, contact tracing, licensing sex workers, and "crimes" of transmission. Analysis is weak in places, but this article is helpful in understanding the general nature of public health legislation.

Guinan, Mary and Ann Hardy, "Epidemiology of AIDS in Women in the United States: 1981 through 1986," *Journal of the American Medical Association*, Vol. 257:15, April 17, 1987.

Basic scientific information, but the analysis gets screwed up. They advocate celibacy, for example. See Wofsy's rejoinder below.

Hammonds, Evelynn, "Race, Sex and AIDS," Radical America, Vol. 20:6, 1986-1987.

Analysis of the impact of AIDS on Black women in the United States, in the special issue of *RA* "Facing AIDS." In the same issue is Dooley Worth and Ruth Rodriguez's "Latina Women and AIDS." Also see Margaret Cerullo and Hammonds' article "AIDS in Africa: The Western Imagination and the Dark Continent," *Radical America*, Vol. 21:2-3, 1987-1988.

Hepburn, Cuca and Bonnie Gutierrez, *Alive and Well: A Lesbian Health Guide*, Trumansburg, NY: Crossing Press, 1988.

Well, by identifying their front-row audience as gold-star dykes, you know, those of us "exclusively involved with women-loving women," Hepburn and Gutierrez avoid dealing much with certain sticky issues. Chapter 5, "Lesbians and AIDS," capitulates to reality, though. Lesbian sexuality is complex, isn't it.

"HIV Infection: Obstetric and Perinatal Issues," *Lancet*, April 9, 1988.

Discusses the effect of AIDS on pregnancy, factors associated with perinatal transmission and counseling HIV-infected pregnant women. Also see

Gloeb, J., "Human Immunodeficiency Virus Infection in Women: The Effects of HIV on Pregnancy," *American Journal of Obstetrics and Gynecology*, Vol. 159:3, September 1988.

Goedert et al., "Mother-to-infant transmission of HIV..." *Lancet*, December 9, 1989.

Koonin, L.M. et al., "Pregnancy-associated Deaths Due to AIDS in the United States," *Journal of the American Medical Association*, Vol. 261:9, March 3, 1989.

Minkoff, H.L., "Care of Pregnant Women Infected with Human Immunodeficiency Virus," *Journal of the American Medical Association*, Vol. 258:19, 1987.

Mitchell, Janet, "What About the Mothers of HIV-Infected Babies?" *National AIDS Network Multi-Cultural Notes on AIDS Education and Service*, Vol. 1:10, April 1988.

"Mother-to-Child Transmission of HIV Infection, The European Collaborative Study," *Lancet*, November 5, 1988.

Selwyn, P.A. et al., "Knowledge of HIV Antibody Status and Decisions to Continue or Terminate Pregnancy Among Intravenous Drug Users," *Journal of the American Medical Association*, Vol. 261:24, June 23, 1989.

Hubbard, Ruth, Mary Sue Henefin, and Barbara Fried, eds., *Women Looking at Biology Looking at Women*, Cambridge, MA: Schenkman, 1979.

A critique of the Western scientific establishment; outlines the role of biology and social science in the denigration and oppression of women. Also see Hubbard's *Biological Woman—The Convenient Myth: A Collection of Feminist Essays and a Comprehensive Bibliography*, Cambridge, MA: Schenkman, 1982, which reprints six articles from the above with new ones on lesbianism, Black women's health, menstruation, and the interaction of culture with biology. Includes an extensive bibliography on women and science.

Hull, Gloria, Patricia Bell Scott, and Barbara Smith, eds., *All the Women Are White, All the Blacks Are Men, But Some of Us Are Brave: Black Women's Studies,* Old Westbury, NY: Feminist Press, 1982.

Essays on feminism, racism, literature, health, education, social science, and religion. Contributors include Michelle Wallace, The Combahee River Collective, Ellen Pence, and Beverly Smith among others.

Kaplan, Helen Singer, *The Real Truth About Women and AIDS,* New York: Simon & Schuster, 1988.

Amazing what passes for truth here. Kaplan would have us all take the antibody test before having sex with members of dreaded risk groups. Either that or not have sex at all. Again, she confuses risk groups with risk behaviors, raising fears about transmission, then dispelling them for heterosexuals. Chances are so slim, you know. And guess what, there's no such thing as woman-to-woman sex. ACT UP's Women's Caucus zapped this little piece of work by adhering warning stickers to copies on bookstore shelves.

Langone, John, *AIDS: The Facts,* Boston: Little Brown, 1988.

Like many other books on the general topic of AIDS, Langone's excludes discussion about how HIV affects women. Langone and Little Brown are remiss in oh so many ways, though. Get this: there's a chapter entitled, "How did the virus go from monkeys to humans."

Lester, Bonnie, *Women and AIDS: A Practical Guide for Those Who Help Others,* New York: Continuum, 1989.

Well, for heaven's sake. For the first volume in Continuum's counseling series, psychologist Lester addresses us solely as caretakers of men. Yes, women do comfort the sick, change the sheets, and cook the food, but we also get AIDS and HIV infection! There is just a tad about how HIV affects women's bodies. Lester bolsters women's role as nurturing others, saying, for example, that women "do not face the stigma of contracting and transmitting the disease through homosexuality."

Lipnack, Jessica, "The Women's Health Movement: A Special Report," *New Age,* Vol. 5:9, March 1980.

Good discussion of this movement's rise and politics.

Lorde, Audre, *The Cancer Journals,* Argyle, NY: Spinsters, Ink, 1980.

Lorde tells the story of her meeting the Western medical establishment. Her insight in this telling is characteristically profound. Also see Lorde's essay "Uses of the Erotic," *Sister Outsider,* Trumansburg, NY: Crossing, 1984.

Marmor, M.L. et al., "Possible Female-to-Female Transmission of Human Immunodeficiency Virus (letter)," *Annals of Internal Medicine,* Vol. 105:969, December 1986.

And still no cunnilingual transmission information from the CDC. For more evidence see

Monzon, O.T. and J.M. Capellan, "Female-to-female transmission of HIV (letter)," *Lancet,* July 4, 1987.

Perry, S. et al., "Orogenital Transmission of Human Immunodeficiency Virus (letter)," *Annals of Internal Medicine,* Vol. 111:11, 1989.

Sabatini, M.T., K. Patel, and R. Hirschman, "Kaposi's Sarcoma and T-Cell Lymphoma in an Immunodeficient Woman: A Case Report," *AIDS Research,* Vol. 1, 1984.

Spitzer, P.G. and N.J. Weiner, "Transmission of HIV Infection From a Woman to a Man by Oral Sex," *New England Journal of Medicine*, Vol. 320:251, 1989.

McCaskell, Lisa, "We Are Not Immune: Women and AIDS," *Healthsharing*, Fall 1988.

Women Healthsharing is a dynamite women's health care journal run collectively in Toronto. This article covers some basic issues around women and HIV: transmission, safer sex for heterosexuals and lesbians, testing, and epidemiology. Darien Taylor's "Testing Positive: Supporting Women With HIV" in the March 1990 issue discusses how and why seropositive women should support each other.

Minkowitz, Donna, "Safe and Sappho: An AIDS Primer for Lesbians," *Village Voice*, February 21, 1988.

Go, Donna. This was the first article in the *Voice* discussing safer sex for lesbians.

Mitchell, C., "Women are W.A.R.N.ed about AIDS," *Wave*, January 28, 1989.

Interviews WARN's Vivian Brown and Debra Mackay about work with sex workers and sex partners of needle sharers in Los Angeles.

Moraga, Cherrie and Gloria Anzaldua, eds., *This Bridge Called My Back: Writings by Radical Women of Color*, New York: Kitchen Table/Women of Color Press, 1981.

This landmark anthology contains analysis, poetry, interviews, and essays that enrich, revise, and shake down feminist thought. Includes Audre Lorde's "The Master's Tools Will Never Dismantle the Master's House" and the Combahee River Collective's "A Black Feminist Statement."

Morin, Jack, *Anal Pleasure and Health: A Guide for Men and Women*, Burlingame, CA: YES Press, 1989.

There should be a slew of new books with this matter-of-fact focus on anal sex, but this title stands virtually alone on bookstore shelves. This stuff is VITAL to know if you partake in butt fucking. It's written well and fun to read.

Murray, Marea, "Battles Joined: Odyssey of a Lesbian AIDS Activist," *Gay Community News*, February - March 1988 (5-part series).

Murray has written lots about AIDS activism and safer lesbian sex in *Gay Community News*, *Bad Attitude*, *On Our Backs*, and *Bay Windows*.

Norwood, Chris, *Advice for Life: A Woman's Guide to AIDS Risks and Prevention, A National Women's Health Network Guide*, New York: Pantheon, 1987.

Norwood realizes that women, not men, need to talk to each other about transmission issues. But her advice here is divisive. She blames prostitutes for heterosexual AIDS, focusing concern for "innocent" women "victimized" by men who've had illicit sex with men or prostitutes. She wants antibody testing to be a public imperative. Norwood says that as long as blood isn't involved, there's "no indication that dental dams are generally needed" when having oral sex with a woman. We may want to use them with an infected partner, she says, to "simply feel safer."

—, "Alarming Rise in Deaths: Are Women Showing New AIDS Symptoms?" *Ms.*, July 1988.

Norwood is right here, though, in noting that the CDC undercounts the number of women who die from HIV-related illnesses because certain diseases are officially ignored. For example, the CDC definition of AIDS fails to include pelvic inflammatory disease (PID), common among HIV-infected women. The CDC defines AIDS by symptoms men exhibit, ignoring those only exhibited by HIV-infected women.

—, "AIDS: The Toll of Apathy," *The Discovery Channel*, February 1990.

Norwood talks to WARN's Marie St. Cyr and ADAPT's Yolanda Serrano for this article. Swinging around to better sense from her *Advice for Life*, she says here that "a tiny (HIV) virus doesn't require an open lesion for infection." So should cunnilinguists use barriers now? Norwood likes the idea of mandatory partner notification, assuming that the state cutting through us like that will really be for our own good in the long run. As Norwood suggests, *Cosmo* should retract the misinformation Dr. Gould presented. She might examine her own thinking about transmission, choice, and volition as well.

O'Malley, Padraiz, ed., *The AIDS Epidemic: Private Rights and the Public Interest*, Boston: Beacon, 1988.

Includes an article "Women and AIDS" by P. Clay Stephens, formerly of Fenway Community Health Center in Boston.

Our Lives in the Balance: U.S. Women of Color and the AIDS Epidemic, Latham, NY: Kitchen Table Women of Color Press, 1991 (forthcoming).

Coeditors Alma Crawford, Val Kanuha, Aleah Long, Veneita Porter, Helen Rodriguez, and Beverly Smith have created the first book presenting responses of women of color to the AIDS/HIV health crisis. Slated to be released sometime in 1990, *Our Lives* features conversations with women PWAs, as well as activists and health care workers discussing the challenges faced and visions created. Text in English and Spanish.

Outweek, 159 West 25th Street, New York, NY 10001, 212/337-1200, Weekly, June 1989-.

This new queer weekly out of New York keeps close tabs on politics, especially ACT UP's. You've heard of "outing"? It started here. They try hard to cover lesbian and women's issues, and they do pretty well, tons better than *The New York Native*. Maybe *Outweek* will get more dykes with serious editorial power on staff soon.

Panos Institute. *AIDS and the Third World*, London: Panos Institute (8 Alfred Place, London, WC1E 7EB, UK or 1409 King St., Alexandria, VA 22314), 1988.

Published in association with the Norwegian Red Cross, this contains statistics on HIV and AIDS cases from Third World countries. It identifies the countries most affected by AIDS (French Guiana, Bermuda, Bahamas, Congo, United States, Guadeloupe, Burundi, Haiti, Barbados, Trinidad—in that order) by using WHO statistics for the number of AIDS cases per million. Suggests African governments are reluctant to reveal the large scale of the AIDS pandemic. The Chirimuutas challenge the statistics and strategy (see above).

Patton, Cindy, *Sex and Germs: The Politics of AIDS*, Boston: South End Press, 1985.

A smart and passionate telling of gay/lesbian grassroots political response to AIDS. Patton, a political activist and health care worker, broke ground with this work that has synthesized and catalyzed gay and lesbian political response to the pandemic. Patton has written intelligently about AIDS and activism from the early days. See especially her work in *Gay Community News*. You also might be interested in the interview with Patton in the April 1989 issue of *Rites* where she talks about porn, safer sex for women, and politics. Also see her piece on the AIDS "industry" in Carter and Watney's

Taking Liberties. Sex and Germs received the American Library Association's 1985 Lesbian and Gay Book Award.

—and Janis Kelly, *Making It: A Woman's Guide to Sex in the Age of AIDS,* Ithaca, NY: Firebrand Books, 1987.

In Spanish (translation by Papusa Molina) and English with illustrations by Allison Bechdel, this is the best, most thorough, explicit, and entertaining guide for doing it more safely, for both heterosexuals and lesbians.

—and Jennifer Walter, "Sexual Choices and Testing," *Sojourner,* July 1987.

Discusses the politics of HIV testing.

Peavey, Fran, *A Shallow Pool of Time: An HIV+ Woman Grapples with the AIDS Epidemic,* Philadelphia: New Society Publishers, 1990.

Peavey, a San Franciscan, shares thoughts about how AIDS and HIV have affected her community and her life.

Petchesky, Rosalind, *Abortion and Woman's Choice: The State, Sexuality, and Reproductive Freedom,* New York: Longman, 1984.

A thorough feminist treatment of the history of reproductive politics, including the history of its practice and the state's evolving efforts to regulate it. Includes a look at CARASA's politics.

Pharr, Suzanne, *Homophobia: A Weapon of Sexism,* Inverness, CA: Chardon Press, 1988.

An analysis of the relationship between the hatred of queers and the hatred of women.

Pheterson, Gail, ed., *A Vindication of the Rights of Whores: The International Movement for Prostitutes' Rights,* Seattle, WA: Seal Press, 1989.

Like *Sex Work,* this is a fine compilation of essays and writings by working women in a well-spun world wide network. The book is based on the proceedings of the International Committee for Prostitutes' Rights European Parliament held in Brussels, October 1986. The voices are clear; the work is excellent.

Pomerantz, Roger, et al., "Human Immunodeficiency Virus (HIV) Infection of the Uterine Cervix," *Annals of Internal Medicine,* Vol. 108:3, March 1988.

Suggests that "HIV enters cervical secretions from selected infected cell populations within the cervical tissue. The HIV-infected cells in cervical tissue may be involved in transmission of HIV by heterosexual contact [sic] and to neonates born to HIV-infected women."

Potler, Cathy, *AIDS in Prison: A Crisis in New York State Corrections,* The Correctional Association of New York (135 E. 15th St., NY, NY 10003), June 1988.

Summarizes findings and recommendations of the Correctional Association, this state's only public interest organization authorized to make recommendations to the legislature.

PWA Coalition Newsline, New York: PWA Coalition, Inc., 31 West 26th St., New York, NY 10010, 212/532-0290.

Published and distributed free in New York by the PWA Coalition, *Newsline* is a forum of letters, essays, and political and treatment updates by and for PWAs. It has a good resource directory. So far, *Newsline* is not as strong as *The Body Politic* on women's issues.

Rhoads, J.L. et al., "Chronic Vaginal Candidiasis in Women with Human Immuno-deficiency Virus Infection," *Journal of the American Medical Association*, Vol. 257:22, June 12, 1987.

HIV-infected women show symptoms different from men. Also see Sillman, F.H. and A. Sedlis, "Anogenital Papillomavirus Infection and Neoplasia in Immunodeficient Women," *Obstetrics and Gynecology Clinics of North America*, Vol. 14:2, June 1987.

Ribble, Denise, "Not Just Another Article on Lesbian Safe Sex," *Sappho's Isle*, July 1989.

Includes a risk assessment survey by a most thoughtful and diligent RN.

Rich, Adrienne, "Compulsory Heterosexuality and Lesbian Existence," *Signs*, Vol. 5:4, Summer 1980.

Compulsory Reading for Everyone's Existence.

Richardson, Diane, *Women and AIDS*, New York: Methuen, 1988.

Richardson is explicit about safer and unsafe sexual practices and methods of drug use. The book includes transmission information involving blood transfusions, rape, artificial insemination, and pregnancy. It has shortcomings; for example, it toys with the green monkey theory concerning the origin of HIV. The text sometimes confuses risk groups with risk behaviors. Includes a good resources list.

Rieder, Ines and Patricia Ruppelt, eds., *AIDS: The Women*. Pittsburgh: Cleis Press, 1988.

Setting out to "give a face, or many faces, to women's involvement and affliction with the AIDS epidemic," Rieder and Ruppelt anthologized essays in various categories: Family, lovers, and friends of PWAs; Women with AIDS/ARC and HIV-positive women; The professional caregivers; Lesbians facing AIDS; Prostitution in the age of AIDS; Women AIDS educators; AIDS prevention policies. Forty-one women contributors come from a range of social, cultural, racial, and sexual backgrounds; all have found their lives entirely transformed by AIDS. Though the anthology offers stories, advice, and analysis, it does not include explicit information about HIV transmission, treatment, or preventative practices.

Rosenberg, Michael and Jodie Weiner, "Prostitutes and AIDS: A Health Department Priority?," *American Journal of Public Health*, Vol. 78:4, 1988.

It is painful to read stuff laced so thickly with sexism. This presents uninformed arguments regarding "targeting female prostitutes" as a "high-priority component" of "AIDS-prevention strategy."

Routte-Gomez, E, "Horizontes takes message about AIDS to S.J. Junkies," *San Juan Star*, January 30, 1989.

Newspaper article about the National Institute on Drug Abuse program for IVDUs in Puerto Rico.

Rubin, Gayle, "The Traffic in Women: Notes on the 'Political Economy' of Sex," *Toward an Anthropology of Women*, ed., Rayna Reiter, New York: Monthly Review Press, 1975.

A lengthy essay on the interdependence of sex, economics, and politics.

Ruzek, Sheryl, *The Women's Health Movement: Feminist Alternatives to Medical Control*, New York: Praeger, 1978.

Feminist analysis of self-help and empowerment, and its potential for revolutionizing the nature of medical care.

Sabatier, Renee, ed., *Blaming Others: Prejudice, Race, and Worldwide AIDS,* Philadelphia: New Society Publishers, 1988.

Black and Hispanic women, Sabatier notes, account for 71 percent of reported AIDS cases among women in the United States. Citing "the epidemic of social, cultural, economic and political reactions to AIDS" as being "as central to the global AIDS challenge as the disease itself," Sabatier's work focuses on AIDS as it intersects with our prevailing perceptions of sex laden with ethnocentrism, racism, and stigmatization.

Santee, Barbara, *Women and AIDS: The Silent Epidemic,* New York: Women and AIDS Resource Network (135 W. 4th St., c/o United Methodist Church, New York, NY 10012), 1988.

A 26-page well-written, clear-headed treatment of the issues. Santee focuses on risk factors/behaviors as opposed to risk groups; includes comparative data on U.S. and New York City transmission rates.

Schulman, Sarah, "AIDS and Homelessness: Thousands May Die in the Streets," *The Nation,* April 10, 1989.

"According to the Partnership for the Homeless, of the more than 90,000 homeless people in New York City, up to 8,000 have AIDS or AIDS-related complex (ARC). To date, the city has provided sixty-six beds for their care." Sarah's journalism is plain and stark and smart and it bites. She's been writing about politics for a long time, mostly in the queer and feminist press. See particularly "The Left and Passionate Homosexuality" in *GCN* May 8, 1988; "Women Need Not Apply: Institutional Discrimination in Drug Trials," *Village Voice,* February 23, 1988; "Lesbians Respond to AIDS Hysteria," *New York Native,* December 2, 1988; "Health or Homophobia: Responses to the Bathhouses," *New York Native,* November, 1985; "AIDS Hysteria Will Change Your Life," *Womanews,* December 1986. She's better known these days as a novelist. Her latest, *People in Trouble,* Dutton, 1990, features a familiar-looking queer/AIDS activist group called Justice.

Shaw, Nancy and Lyn Paleo, "Women and AIDS," *What To Do About AIDS,* ed., Leon McKusick, Berkeley: University of California Press, 1986.

Shaw and Paleo discuss the nature and politics of epidemiology, pregnancy, pediatric issues, and "levels of risk." They point out that, contrary to popular belief, "there is no evidence that prostitutes constitute a special risk category" for HIV infection.

SIECUS Report, Sex Information Education Council of the United States, 32 Washington Place, New York, NY 10003, 212/673-3850.

SIECUS was founded in 1964 to establish sex as a "healthy entity" in the American psyche. Now loosely affiliated with New York University, SIECUS continues to produce this bimonthly publication well worth more readership than it currently attracts. They've also got a nifty library you can arrange to visit if you want. See especially

"Cultural Diversity and Sexuality/AIDS Information and Education," February/March 1990 (focuses on Latin, Native American, and Asian & Pacific Islander communities).

"Sexuality Education," December 1989/January 1990.

"The Truth About Condoms," November/December 1988.

"Adolescent Sexuality and Abstinence," September/October 1988: "AIDS Prevention and Civil Liberties: the False Security of Mandatory Testing," May/June 1987.

"Latino Culture and Sex Education," and January/February 1987 (with Dooley Worth and Ruth Rodriguez' "Latina Women and AIDS").

Slaughter, R, "Responding to the AIDS Crisis: The Challenge to Shelters," *The Exchange: A Forum on Domestic Violence,* Fall/Winter 1989.

Slaughter is with the WARN project in Los Angeles, here emphasizing the crucial role shelter staff could have in meaningful AIDS education.

Snitow, Ann, Christine Stansell, and Sharon Thompson, eds., *Powers of Desire: The Politics of Sexuality,* New York: Monthly Review Press, 1983.

Includes a range of contributions by lesbian, gay, and heterosexual women writers about the histories and class/race/sex politics of female sexuality. Most of the essays were published elsewhere first, so the anthology contains a selected range of "representative" work important to sex lib politics today.

Starr, Paul, *The Social Transformation of American Medicine,* New York: Basic Books, 1982.

This book got a lot of hype in academic circles when it came out. It's a neat little cultural analysis of the development of the empire.

Sturdevant, Saundra, "The Military, Women and AIDS: The Bar Girls of Subic Bay," *The Nation,* April 3, 1989.

Subtitle should be "The Military Boys of Subic Bay." It's about the typically gross irresponsibility of U.S. military men and boys regarding HIV transmission and related issues. Also read Freda Guttman's, "Daughters of the Dispossessed: Prostitution in the Philippines," in *Healthsharing,* Summer 1986.

U.S. Department of Health and Human Services, Public Health Service, Centers for Disease Control, Center for Infectious Diseases, Division of HIV/AIDS. *HIV/AIDS Surveillance.*

We all know the government can't count, but you can get this 15-page monthly report mailed to you free for your own analysis. To get on the mailing list write: Centers for Disease Control, Division of HIV/AIDS, Technical Information Activity, Mailstop G-29, Atlanta, GA 30333. Otherwise, you can find it in almost any library that participates in the Federal Depository Library Program. Or you can call the CDC's National AIDS Information Clearinghouse (NAIC) for the most up-to-date HIV/AIDS stats: just call 301/762-5111. The 13 or so statistical sets in this report include: "AIDS cases by age group, exposure category, and sex," "AIDS cases by sex, exposure category, and race/ethnicity," and "Results of investigations of adult/adolescent AIDS cases with undetermined risk." An expanded, year-end edition is published each January. In addition, municipal departments of health may publish local AIDS/HIV statistics. The New York City Department of Health AIDS Surveillance Unit publishes monthly reports; write: 346 Broadway, Rm. 706, New York, NY 10013, 212/566-7561.

U.S. Department of Health and Human Services, Public Health Service, National Center for Health Services Research and Health Care Technology Assessment. *NCHSR Program Note: Selected Bibliography on AIDS for Health Services Research,* September 1989. 18 -12 Parklawn Bldg., Rockville, MD 20857, 301/443-4100.

Well, you can bet there isn't much overlap between the NCHSR bibliography and this one here. This NCHSR bibliography has 256 annotated cites in it from August 1988-August 1989. It supplements two previous bibliographies published in September 1987 and 1988. It cites only mainstream

Western scientific and public health journals. In the subject index, there are no citations under "women"! There are three cites under "pregnant women" and four under "prostitutes," though. Oh, of course, there we are. If you look hard enough, you might find some other relevant stuff, maybe in the epidemiology section.

U.S. Department of Health and Human Services, Public Health Service, National Institutes of Health, National Library of Medicine, *AIDS Bibliography,* 8600 Rockville Pike, Bethesda, MD 20894.

This is the paper copy version of the database AIDSLINE, a subset of the MEDLINE database. The paper copy sells from the Government Printing Office for $43/year, so most libraries can afford it. Journals indexed all represent mainstream medical and public policy interests. The bibliography is extraordinarily weak on women, especially the paper version. In the database, which is available through Dialog, at least there are several headings for each cite, one of which is likely to be "women" or "female" or "pregnancy" or "prostitutes" or something possibly sexist but at least you can find it. But in the paper copy, there's only one subject word for each citation. So, in the September 1989 issue there are ZERO cites under "women," but six under "pregnancy complications, infections," and two under "prostitution." One more thing, notice how the government sponsors indexing of all this kind of mainstream lit, but there is no indexing for *Womanews* or *On Our Backs;* you have to dig through crumbling newsprint if you want to find stuff there. *Alternative Press Index* does some for us, but do they have a database? NO WAY. Knowledge is power. Just one more example of how we're uncmpowered by our government.

U.S. Public Health Service, *Women and AIDS: Initiatives of the Public Health Service. A Report of the PHS Coordinating Committee on Women's Health Issues.* 1987.

In a now-dated document that's more damning than not, this is a compilation of reports from agencies including the CDC, FDA, and NIH regarding programs and support for women with AIDS.

Vance, Carol, ed., *Pleasure and Danger: Exploring Female Sexuality,* London: Routledge and Kegan Paul, 1984.

A popular anthology containing essays on a variety of socio-, psycho-, sexual issues from more than 30 contributors. A good companion piece of work to Snitow annotated above.

Wallace, Joyce, "AIDS in Prostitutes," *AIDS and Infections of Homosexual Men,* Pearl Ma and Donald Armstrong, eds., Boston: Butterworths, 1989.

Contains a brief account of the only study of johns' seroprevalance to date.

Walter, Melitta, ed., *Ach war's doch nur ein boser Traum! Frauen und AIDS,* Freiburg: Kore Verlag (Holbeinstrasse 12, D-7800 Freiburg i. Br., West Germany), 1987.

Translation: If It Were Only A Bad Dream! Women and AIDS.

Watney, Simon, "Missionary Positions: AIDS, 'Africa,' and Race," *Differences,* Winter 1989.

Watney's essay challenges sexist, racist notions about "African AIDS," calling up language from Conrad's *Heart of Darkness* and comparing it to current ideas about "the infectious continent." Also see Watney's better known book *Policing Desire: Pornography, AIDS & the Media,* Minneapolis: University of Minnesota Press, 1987.

Watstein, Sarah Barbara and Robert Anthony Laurich, *Women and AIDS: A Sourcebook,* Phoenix, AZ: Oryx Press, 1990.

More librarians tackle women and AIDS info.

White, Evelyn, ed., *The Black Women's Health Book: Speaking for Ourselves,* Seattle: Seal Press, 1990.

Byllye Avery, founder of the National Black Women's Health Project based in Atlanta, explains in a *Gay Community News* interview that this book "is a heartfelt protest against the racism that cripples the medical establishment and consequently our lives." The 41 contributors to the anthology have rendered a spectrum of Black women's experiences with health care using personal, professional, poetic, and scholarly accounts. This is fine feminist work, including voices of women from different eras, classes, and sexual backgrounds.

Winnow, Jackie. "Lesbians Working on AIDS: Assessing the Impact on Health Care for Women," *Out/Look,* Summer 1989.

Assembles a number of reasons why we're here.

Wofsy, Constance, "Human Immunodeficiency Virus Infection in Women," *Journal of the American Medical Association,* Vol. 257:15, April 17, 1987.

A clear-sighted editorial checking Guinan and Hardy's work in the same issue. For a lengthier exposition, see Wofsy's "Women and the Acquired Immunodeficiency Syndrome: An Interview," *Western Journal of Medicine,* Vol. 149:6, December 1988.

Women and AIDS, San Francisco AIDS Foundation, 1989, 1-800-342-AIDS.

The foundation's primary pamphlet for women addresses pregnancy, breast-feeding, and artificial insemination. Text by Women's AIDS Network. Also see the pamphlets *Lesbians and AIDS, Pregnancy and AIDS, AIDS Kills Women and Children,* and *Condoms for Couples.* The SFAF catalog says there's a $100 minimum on all orders of educational material, but you can order a sampler packet for five dollars.

Women and AIDS: An Annotated Bibliography for Project Staff and Clients. NOVA Research Company (4600 East-West Highway, Suite 700, Bethesda, MD 20814, 301/986-1891), 6th Edition, December 1989.

A substantial bibliography (229 pages) prepared for the National Institute on Drug Abuse. Contains entries from scientific and social service journals and some popular and political magazines. Annotations are thorough. Call or write to receive a free copy.

Women and AIDS: Clinical Resource Guide, San Francisco AIDS Foundation (333 Valencia St., P.O. Box 6182, San Francisco, CA 94101-6182, 415/861-3397), 1987.

This is a great collection of resource listings and medical and social service articles. It's a little dated, but it may be revived one of these days.

AIDS Videos By, For, and About Women

CATHERINE SAALFIELD

Video is among the most useful tools available to AIDS activists and educators. In fact, a veritable video revolution has taken place around the subject of AIDS in the United States as well as in numerous other countries, relative to the availability of television facilities and consumer format video equipment. AIDS tapes vary widely in originality, accuracy, and cultural sensitivity, differing in every way possible. New tapes are produced almost daily, ranging from 15-second public service announcements to two-hour documentaries and dramas.

Following is a list of videotapes pertaining to women and AIDS. In no way comprehensive, this list is meant to inspire the reader to seek out these and other tapes for your own use—to buy, borrow, or rent to watch at home if you have your own VCR—and for use by organizations in your community. These tapes can be screened in any number of public situations, including on broadcast, cable, or public access TV, or in hospitals, health clinics, community centers, service centers, prisons, waiting rooms, schools, fundraising situations, and activist organizations.

Each entry lists the tape's title, director, city where the tape was produced, name of individual or organization who produced the tape, date, and a brief description; at the end of each entry the distributor's name is noted in brackets. A list of distributors follows the list of annotated selections. Many distribute numerous AIDS tapes even if only one or two are referred to in this list. All videotapes are in English unless otherwise noted.

Some private and city-funded organizations have created "lending libraries" to facilitate community access to AIDS videos. For example, in New York City, the Library for AIDS Resources, in the NYC Department of Health, has a video lending library open to health professionals and community-based AIDS service providers. Because of limited resources, the library must be called for an appointment (212/566-1800, 1801). All of their services are free, and they have a video guide listing their available tapes (Library for AIDS Resources, 125 Worth Street, Box A-1, New York, NY 10013). They can also be reached from out of state for resources in other cities, like the AIDS Library of Philadelphia and a similar program in Los Angeles. For further information about AIDS media and an updated general guide listing films and videotapes about AIDS, contact Media Network, 121 Fulton Street, 5th floor, New York, NY 10038, 212/619-3455. Their resources were instrumental in putting together this list.

AIDS and the Women's Community. San Francisco AIDS Foundation/Bay Area Career Women, 1986. 44 min. An in-depth view of the impact AIDS has had on the lesbian community in San Francisco, addressing risk factors, transmission, safe sex, emotional issues, and political aspects of the crisis. [San Francisco AIDS Foundation (SFAF)]

AIDS in the Barrio. Peter Biella and Frances Negron. Philadelphia: Alba Martinez and Frances Negron, producers; David Haas, executive producer; 1989. Film, available in video, 30 min., Spanish with English subtitles. Documents the impact of AIDS on one Latino community. Especially strong interviews with women about being the sexual partners of intravenous drug users (IVDUs) and about sexism in their lives. Does not include information on transmission or prevention; lacks gay characters. [AIDS Film Initiative]

AIDS Is about Secrets. Sandra Elkin. New York: HIV Center for Clinical and Behavioral Studies, 1989. 37 min. A soap opera-style tape targeted at Black women who are sex partners of IVDUs. Represents the real life situations of four women, by dramatizing the behaviors that place them at risk. [Clare Walsh Associates]

AIDS: Me and My Baby. New York: HIV Center for Clinical and Behavioral Studies, 1988. 23 min. Sandra Elkin. Similar in style to *AIDS Is about Secrets.* Targeted at Black and Latino communities, and primarily at heterosexuals. Unfortunately, gay people pictured only in prison. [Clare Walsh Associates]

Angry Initiatives, Defiant Strategies: Deep Dish AIDS Show. John Greyson, coordinator. New York: Deep Dish TV, 1987. 60 min. A compilation of excerpts from 32 grassroots video productions from throughout the country about AIDS. Hosted by caricatures of Liz Taylor and Liberace. [Deep Dish TV]

Are You with Me? M. Neema Barnette. New York: AIDSFILMS, 1989. 17 min. Dramatizes when a divorced mother encourages her teenage daughter to take precautions in her relationship with a man, but finds it hard to practice what she preaches. [AIDSFILMS]

Bleach, Teach and Outreach. Catherine Saalfield and Ray Navarro. New York: Gay Men's Health Crisis (GMHC), 1988. 28 min. Focuses on the highly controversial implementation of the Needle Exchange and Education Program by the New York City Department of Health. Demonstrates the integral role of the Association of Drug Abuse Prevention and Treatment (ADAPT) in originating and fulfilling this program. Illustrates the community-based struggle for a way to curb the transmission of HIV among IVDUs. [GMHC]

Clips. Debbie Sundhal and Nan Kinney. San Francisco: Femme Fatale Video, 1989. 30 min. Safe-sex porn for lesbians, in three ten-minute vignettes. Includes the celebrated female ejaculation short. [Blush Entertainment]

Current Flow. New York: GMHC, 1989. 4 min. An erotic safer-sex tape for women who have sex with other women. One in a series of safer-sex shorts. [GMHC]

DiAna's Hair Ego: AIDS Info Up Front. Ellen Spiro, 1989. 30 min. Focuses on DiAna DiAna, who began as an AIDS educator by handing out condoms to customers in her beauty shop in Columbia, S.C. She and partner Dr. Bambi Sumpter now run the South Carolina AIDS Education Network (SCAEN) on the shop's tips because the state AIDS agency refuses to support their upfront style of confronting the issues. [Video Data Bank]

Doctors, Liars and Women: AIDS Activists Say No to Cosmo. Jean Carlomusto and Maria Maggenti. New York: GMHC, 1988. 23 min. Documents the actions of the Women's Caucus of ACT UP. Analyzes and protests the lies behind a murderous *Cosmopolitan* article that misled women about HIV transmission and unprotected heterosexual sex. [GMHC]

Drugs and AIDS: Getting the Message Out. Washington, DC: State of the Art, Inc., 1988. 30 min. A how-to tape for the IV drug-using community. Includes how to get help: programs, pamphlets, prophylaxis. [WETA Educational Activities]

Dying for Love. Shari Cookson, Burlington, VT: Lifetime Cable Network, 1987. 50 min. Profiles four women living with AIDS. An excellent tape: multiracial, geographically diverse, and gay positive. [Lifetime Television]

Family Values. David Stuart, San Francisco, 1989. 58 min. Includes excellent testimony. Documents the supportive and loving response of San Francisco lesbian community to the AIDS crisis. [Hands On Productions]

He Left Me His Strength. Sherry Busbee and Merle Jawitz. New York: Busbee, Jawitz, Sheila Ward, and John Bassinger, 1989. 13 min. Portrays the inspirational role of Mildred Pearson, whose son died of AIDS-related complications, in AIDS education and activism for communities of color. [April Productions]

Her Giveaway. Mona Smith. Minneapolis: Renee White Rabbit, 1988. 30 min. Native American Carol Lafavor intimately discusses the realities of being a woman with AIDS and her holistic approach to her own illness. [Minnesota Indian Affairs Council and Women Make Movies]

Julie. Seth Levin, Minneapolis, 1989. 7 min. Uses Julie's journal entries to document the daily life of an empowered woman with AIDS. [Twin Cities Public Television]

Latex and Lace. Laird Sutton, Janet Taylor, and Dolores Bishop. San Francisco: Exodus Trust, 1988. 22 min. Explicit safer-sex tape, in which lesbians and straight and bisexual women talk about AIDS. Also a women-only "safer-sex party." [Multi-Focus]

Living with AIDS: Women and AIDS. Alexandra Juhasz and Jean Carlomusto. New York: GMHC, 1988. 28 min. Fills an enormous gap in material by, for, and about women with AIDS. Counters the inaccuracies and ignorance in the media and the government about HIV-infected women in the United States. [GMHC]

Mildred Pearson: When You Love a Person. Brooklyn, NY: Yannick Durand and the Brooklyn AIDS Task Force, 1988. 9 min. Home video style of photographs with voice-over. Follows one woman's fight for her son's life. Inspiring in her constant and unconditional support of him. [Brooklyn AIDS Task Force]

Prostitutes, Risk and AIDS. Alexandra Juhasz and Jean Carlomusto. New York: GMHC, 1988. 28 min. Examines the scapegoating of prostitutes for HIV/AIDS and sexually transmitted diseases (STDs) among heterosexuals. Also analyzes the media's distortion of the image of who is really at risk for HIV infection. [GMHC]

Reframing AIDS. Pratibha Parmar, London, 1987. 30 min. A series of diverse talking-head-style interviews. Repositions the representations of AIDS in Britain in relation to race, gender, class, and sexual orientation. [Video Data Bank]

Safe Sex Slut. Carol Leigh, San Francisco, 1988. 3 min. Leigh, also known as Scarlot Harlot, is an advocate for prostitutes' rights, an AIDS activist, and a member of the prostitutes' rights group COYOTE (Call Off Your Old Tired Ethics). She produced and stars in this fun music video about safer sex. [Video Data Bank]

Se Met Ko. Patricia Benoit. New York: Haitian Women's Program, 1989. 16mm film, available in video, 28 min., in Creole with English subtitles. Telenovella style. Produced by and for the Haitian community. Portrays charismatic and believable characters who are dealing with the realities of AIDS in their own community. Does not address issues of homophobia/heterosexism or IV drug use. [American Friends Service Committee]

The Second Epidemic. Amber Hollibaugh. New York: Human Rights Commission, 1989. 27 min. A series of video portraits of people living with AIDS who have fought discrimination with the help of the AIDS Discrimination Unit of the Human Rights Commission. An outstanding section on Margie Rivera, a young Puerto Rican woman in New York City. [AIDS Discrimination Unit]

SIDA y Su Familia. Dallas County Health Department, 1988. 12 min., available in Spanish and English, Spanish transcripts available. Very straightforward language. Aimed at both teenagers and adults. Addresses IV drug use, homosexuality, bisexuality, and condom use. [Dallas County Health Department]

So Sad, So Sorry, So What. Jane Gilloolly, Boston, MA, 1990. 27 min. This tape collages still photographs of a young incarcerated woman who discovered she is seropositive when she was jailed. She talks very personally about her life and her illness and the prejudices she faces in the prison around HIV issues and out on the street around issues of drug use. [Fanlight]

Target City Hall. DIVA TV, New York, 1989. 28 min. The first tape by Damned Interfering Video Activist Television (DIVA TV, an affinity group of ACT UP/NY). Includes a wide range of statements on ACT UP's massive demonstration at City Hall on March 28, 1989. The final section, LAPIT (Lesbian Activists Producing Innovative Television), emphasizes the role of women in ACT UP and the media hype around their being illegally strip-searched in jail. [DIVA TV]

A Test for the Nation. Alexandra Juhasz. New York: GMHC, 1988. 25 min. Well-edited video presenting interviews with doctors with various points of view about AIDS and abortion rights. Addresses the coercion of HIV-positive women into having abortions. [GMHC]

Testing the Limits Guide to Safer Sex. Testing the Limits Collective, New York, 1990. 30 min. Engaging and straightforward instruction on safer-sex techniques and how to negotiate safer sex with a partner, by Community Health Project nurse Denise Ribble. Good for all communities. [Testing the Limits]

Testing the Limits: NYC (Part One). New York: Testing the Limits Collective, 1987. 28 min. The first in a series of documentaries about the efforts of grassroots AIDS activists as they organize around the epidemic in New York City. [Testing the Limits]

VIDA. Lourdes Portillo. New York: AIDSFILMS, 1989. 18 min., available in English and Spanish. Dramatizes the story of Elsie, a Latina, single, working mother who finds herself torn between her fear of AIDS and her feelings for the new man in her life. Demonstrates the powerful role women play in setting norms for sexual behavior. [AIDSFILMS]

Women and AIDS: A Survival Kit. Santa Cruz, CA: California AIDS Clearinghouse, 1988. 22 min. Two women with AIDS talk candidly about themselves, transmission issues, safe sex, and use of condoms. [California AIDS Clearinghouse]

Women, Children and AIDS. Jane Wagner, San Francisco, 1987. 30 min. Documents the findings of California-based research projects about women, children, and AIDS. Addresses antibody testing, alternative insemination, drug use, heterosexual transmission, mother-child transmission, psychosocial and health care needs, blood recipients and children at risk. [San Francisco AIDS Foundation]

Distributors

AIDS Discrimination Unit, Human Rights Commission
52 Duane Street, New York, NY 10007
212/566-5177

AIDS Film Initiative
732 West Nedro Avenue, Philadelphia, PA 19120
215/224-4934

AIDSFILMS
50 West 34th Street, #6B6, New York, NY 10001
212/629-6288

American Friends Service Committee Information Services
15 Rutherford Place, New York, NY 10003
212/598-0972

April Productions
236 East 5th Street, New York, NY 10003
212/473-3143

Blush Entertainment
526 Castro Street, San Francisco, CA 94109
415/861-4723

Brooklyn AIDS Task Force
22 Chapel Street, Brooklyn, NY 11201
718/596-4783

California AIDS Clearinghouse
P.O. Box 1830, Santa Cruz, CA 95061
800/258-9090

Clare Walsh Associates
22 Florida Avenue, Staten Island, NY 10305
718/720-4488

Dallas County Health Department
1936 Amelia Court, Dallas, TX 75235
214/920-7916

Deep Dish TV
339 Lafayette Street, New York, NY 10012
212/473-8933

DIVA TV
c/o ACT UP/New York, 496A Hudson Street, #G4, New York, NY 10014
212/989-1114

Fanlight
47 Halifax Street, Boston, MA 02130
617/524-0980

Gay Men's Health Crisis [GMHC]
Videotapes/Publications Distribution
129 West 20th Street, New York, NY 10011
212/337-3558

Hands On Productions
633 Post Street, #500, San Francisco, CA 94109

Lifetime Television
c/o Resolution Video, 1 Mill Street, Burlington, VT 05401

Minnesota Indian Affairs Council: AIDS Taskforce
127 University, St. Paul, MN 55155
612/296-3611

Multi-Focus, Inc.
1525 Franklin Street, San Francisco, CA 94109
415/673-5100

San Francisco AIDS Foundation
333 Valencia Street/P.O. Box 6182, San Francisco, CA 94101
415/861-3397

Testing the Limits Collective
31 West 26th Street, 4th floor, New York, NY 10010
212/545-7120

Twin Cities Public Television
172 East 4th Street, St. Paul, MN 55101
612/222-1717

Video Data Bank
The School of the Art Institute of Chicago
37 South Wabash Avenue, Chicago, IL 60603
312/443-3793

WETA Educational Activities
P.O. Box 2626, Washington, DC 20013
800/445-1964

Women Make Movies
225 Lafayette Street, Suite 207-8, New York, NY 10012
212/925-0606

Index

A

Ableism, 12, 228
Abortion, 13, 79, 93, 104, 105, 159, 160, 162, 200-208, 236
Abscess, 72
Acupuncture, 23, 77, 126
Acyclovir, 71
ADAPT (Association for Drug Abuse Prevention and Treatment), 125, 126, 128, 212
Addiction/Drug Dependence, 72, 123-129, 167, 188
Adolescents, see Teenagers
African, 1, 2, 36, 182
African-American, see also Black, 95, 103-106, 201, 202, 227, 229
Ageism, 178, 228
AIDS Clinical Trial Group (ACTG), 73, 74
AIDS Clinical Trials Information Service, 168
AIDS Counseling and Education (ACE), 141-155
AIDS Coalition to Unleash Power (ACT UP), vii, 66, 82, 119, 137, 171, 205, 212, 215-217, 220, 225, 233, 235-237
AIDS-Related Complex (ARC), 32, 40, 45, 49, 61, 134, 140
Alaskans, 108
Alcohol, 17, 74, 77, 91, 92, 94, 161
Allergic Reactions, 20, 75

Alpha-Interferon, 75
Alternative Insemination, 11, 114
American Civil Liberties Union (ACLU), 65
Americans with Disabilities Act, 65
AmFAR (American Foundation for AIDS Research), 74
Amphetamines, 123
Amphotericin B, 75
Ampligen, 75
Anal Sex, 21, 36, 114, 152, 181
Anemia, 71, 75
Anus, 20, 21, 22, 23, 40, 115
Arthritis, 47
Asian, 3, 32, 107-111, 202
Asthma, 72
Ayurvedic Medicine, 77
AZT, 7, 46, 47, 57, 71, 74, 75, 140, 168, 169, 206

B

Babies, see Infants
Bactrim (Septra), 50, 75, 169, 170
Barbituates, 123
Bedford Hills Correctional Facility, 150, 153
Beta-2 Microglobin, 70, 71
Birth Control/Contraception (IUD, The Pill), 8, 18, 73, 110, 137, 161, 189, 191, 200, 202, 203, 204, 207

Bisexuals, 2, 3, 4, 11, 18, 92, 103,
114, 122, 134, 179, 193-198,
202, 233
Black, see also African-American,
3, 7, 9, 10, 32, 81, 134, 151,
152, 153, 154, 162, 182, 219,
220, 228, 236
Bleach, 23, 127, 141, 147, 180, 184
Bovine Milk Immunogloblin, 76
Breast-feeding, 162, 163
Brooklyn AIDS Task Force
(BATF), 85, 87-89, 150, 232

C

Caesarean Section (C-Section),
162
Cancer, 1, 3, 29, 33, 37, 39, 40, 75,
81, 169, 188, 203
Candida, see also Monilia, Yeast,
34, 40
Canker Sores, 35
CARASA (Committee for Abortion
Rights and Against Sterilization
Abuse), 201
Caribbean, 2, 36, 85, 103-106
CDC (Centers for Disease
Control), 1-3, 32-33, 61, 62, 72,
93, 99, 105, 108, 113-116, 124,
137, 159, 165-166, 217
Cellulitis, 72
Cervical Dysplasia, 36
Cervicitis, 36-37
Chancroid, 19, 34, 36
Chemotherapy, 169
Childbirth, 200
Child Care, 3, 7, 31, 73, 74, 78, 79,
126, 167, 201, 202, 206, 211,
221
Child Custody, 7, 65
Children, 38, 73, 74, 78, 86, 97,
151, 153, 159, 160, 162, 163,
165-172, 174-175, 201, 202,
205, 224, 231
Orphans and Foster Children,
170
Chinese Medicine, 77

Chlamydia, 19, 21, 34, 38, 39, 40,
116, 161, 187, 217
Civil Disobedience, 212, 213, 218
Classism, 9, 10-11, 178, 199, 201
Clinical Markers, 57, 70, 71
Clinoril, 50
Clitoris, 19, 203
Cocaine/Crack, 23, 45, 72, 77,
105, 123, 129, 131, 179
Coccidiodomycosis, 38
Compound Q (Trichosanthin),
11, 76, 208
Condom, 18, 21-22, 28-29, 61, 62,
87, 88, 100, 116-117, 121, 127,
136-137, 141, 147-148, 152,
153, 179-180, 182, 183, 184,
188-189, 191, 195, 197, 204,
212, 216, 219, 222, 228
Condyloma (Warts), 34, 36
Contact Tracing, 64
Contraception, see Birth Control
COYOTE (Call Off Your Old
Tired Ethics), 180, 182
Crack, see Cocaine
Cryptococcal Meningitis, 75
Cryptococcus, 38
Cryptosporidiosis, 38
Cunnilingus, see also Oral Sex,
20, 22, 115, 116
Cytomegalovirus (CMV), 38, 40,
41
Retinitis, 76

D

ddI, 76
Dementia, 3, 37
Demonstrations, see also Civil
Disobedience, 212-214, 216,
220
Dental Dam, 19-23, 28, 61, 116,
121-122, 137, 141, 157, 197,
204, 216-217, 222, 228
Depression, 175
DES, 205, 207
Dextran Sulfate, 76
DHEA, 76

Homophobia, see also
  Heterosexism, 12, 113, 117,
  211, 228, 233, 236
Homosexual, 2-3, 60, 62, 63, 87,
  92, 99, 103, 109, 110
Human Papillomavirus, 33, 37,
  39, 40, 217
Hyde Amendment, 162, 203, 236
Hyperacin (St. John's Wort), 76

I

Immigration/Immigrants, 60, 87,
  108, 109
Immunomodulator, 74, 75
Imreg-1, 77
Incest, 227
Infants/Babies, 60, 62, 73, 159,
  165, 169, 170, 228
  Mortality, 81, 101, 170
Infertility/Fertility, 74, 161
Influenza, 33, 71, 75, 228
Informed Consent, 61, 71, 78, 79,
  141, 207
Insomnia, 35
Interuterine Device (IUD), see
  Birth Control
Intravenous Drug Users (IVDUs),
  2-3, 11, 32, 33, 41, 45, 56, 60,
  63, 66, 72, 73, 92, 95, 99, 101,
  114, 115, 123-129, 143, 151,
  161, 162, 178, 179, 180, 181,
  193, 197, 202
Intravenous (IV) Drugs, 19, 23,
  45, 119, 139, 242
Isosporiasis, 38

J

Jamaican, 85

K

Kaposi's Sarcoma (KS), 29, 38, 53,
  75

L

Lambda Legal Defense and
  Education Fund, 60, 65
Latex, 20-23, 28-29, 64, 116, 137,
  184, 195
Latina/Latino, see also Hispanic,
  1, 3, 5, 7, 32, 81, 99-101, 151,
  153, 236
Lentinan, 77
Lesbian(s), 2, 8, 9, 11, 18, 19, 20,
  22, 27, 31, 36, 66, 86, 109,
  113-118, 119, 136, 193,
  195-198, 200, 202, 212, 216,
  223, 235, 236
Lesbian Herstory Archives, 234
Liver Disease, 72
Loss of Appetite, 35
Lymphadenopathy, 40
Lymphocytes, 70
Lymphogranuloma Venerium, 36
Lymphoma, 38

M

Macrobiotics, 30, 77
MAI, 38
Marijuana, 123
Masturbation, 19, 202
Medicaid, 47, 49, 52, 78, 82, 162,
  166, 168, 177, 203, 233, 236
Megace, 77, 208
Meningitis, 37, 75, 96
Menstrual, see also Period, 17, 21,
  34, 116
Methadone, 45, 70, 126, 132, 161
Miscarriages, 161
Monilia, 34, 38, 39
Mothers, 45, 49, 165-171
Mouth Sores, 35

N

Narcotics Anonymous (NA), 126,
  133
National Abortion Rights Action
  League (NARAL), 201, 204

About South End Press

South End Press is a nonprofit, collectively run book publisher with over 150 titles in print. Since our founding in 1977, we have tried to meet the needs of readers who are exploring, or are already committed to, the politics of radical social change.

Our goal is to publish books that encourage critical thinking and constructive action on the key political, cultural, social, economic, and ecological issues shaping life in the United States and in the world. In this way, we hope to give expression to a wide diversity of democratic social movements and to provide an alternative to the products of corporate publishing.

If you would like a free catalog of South End Press books or information about our membership program—which offers two free books and a 40% discount on all titles—please write us at South End Press, 116 Saint Botolph Street, Boston, MA 02115.

Other titles of interest from South End Press:

Sex and Germs: The Politics of AIDS
Cindy Patton

From Abortion to Reproductive Freedom:
Transforming a Movement
Marlene Gerber Fried, editor

Abortion without Apology:
Radical History for the 1990s
Ninia Baehr

Women Under Attack:
Victories, Backlash, and the Fight for Reproductive Freedom
CARASA (Committee for Abortion Rights and Against Sterilization Abuse),
Susan Davis, editor

Yearning: Race, Gender, and Cultural Politics
bell hooks

Regulating the Lives of Women:
Social Welfare Policy from Colonial Times to the Present
Mimi Abramovitz